To Norma Watson
Best wishes

Matteo Minims

September 1991

Clinical Measurement in Drug Evaluation

Edited by
Walter S. Nimmo, BSc, MD, FRCP, FFARCS, FFARACS
Medical Director
Inveresk Clinical Research, Edinburgh
and Fellow in Anaesthesia
University of Edinburgh
Scotland

Geoffrey T. Tucker, BPharm, PhD
Professor of Clinical Pharmacology
Department of Medicine and Pharmacology
University of Sheffield
England

First ICR International Symposium

Wolfe Publishing Ltd

Copyright © 1991 Wolfe Publishing Ltd
Published by Wolfe Publishing Ltd, 1991
Typeset by Goodfellow & Egan Ltd, Cambridge
Printed by BPCC Hazell Books, Aylesbury, England
ISBN 0 7234 1682 6

A CIP catalogue record for this book is available from the
British Library.

For full details of all Wolfe titles please write to
Wolfe Publishing Ltd, Brook House, 2–16 Torrington Place,
London, WC1E 7LT, England.

Contents

Preface

The measurement of the therapeutic and adverse effects of a drug in humans is a vitally important part of drug evaluation. Very often, more attention is given to measurement of blood concentrations rather than to the effect and this may limit the calculation of dosage regimens which will maximise efficacy and minimise toxicity.

Methods of measurement of drug effects must be reliable, accurate, sensitive, specific and reproducible. In addition, they must be acceptable to patients, clinicians and scientists.

This volume records the proceedings of a symposium held in Edinburgh in May 1990 devoted to the principles and practice of the measurement of drug effects in humans, and its role in the evaluation and development of new drugs. There was emphasis on clinical interpretation and relevance of data as well as the acceptability and accuracy of the methodology. Although stress was placed on the special problems of the cardiovascular and the central nervous systems, all physiological systems were considered. Attention was also given to computer technology, adverse events and special populations.

The symposium was supported by Inveresk Clinical Research and the Scottish Development Agency. We are grateful to members of staff who worked hard to make it successful, especially Louis Campbell-Blair who was responsible for the local organisation. Dr Anthony Pottage of the Astra Clinical Research Unit in Edinburgh and Dr Harry Draffan of Inveresk Research International helped us design the scientific programme, and we record our thanks to them. Most of all, we are indebted to the panel of distinguished speakers from academia and the pharmaceutical industry who agreed to participate and who provided such excellent contributions. Their approach to difficult areas and problematic clinical situations makes their work relevant to everyone who is involved in drug development.

We hope that this volume reminds the delegates of two happy days spent in Edinburgh and encourages scientists to give as much attention as possible to the measurement of drug effects in clinical research.

Walter Nimmo, Edinburgh, and
Geoffrey Tucker, Sheffield

List of Contributors

R. Bergstrand, MD, PhD, Department of Clinical Pharmacology, Astra Hässle AB, Mölndal, Sweden.

A. Breckenridge, MD, MSc, FRCP, Department of Pharmacology and Therapeutics, University of Liverpool, Liverpool, England.

R.W.F. Campbell, MBChB, FRCP, Academic Department of Cardiology, Freeman Hospital, Newcastle-Upon-Tyne, England

R.D. Combes, BSc, PhD, FIBiol, Inveresk Research International, Tranent, Scotland.

H.J. Dargie, MBChB, FRCP, Department of Cardiology, Western Infirmary, Glasgow, Scotland.

P. Demol, MD, Department of Medical Research, Bayer Pharma, Paris, France.

R.F. Drucker, MA, MBBChir, The Upjohn Company, Kalamazoo, MT, USA.

B. Edgar, Dr Med Sci, PhD, Department of Clinical Pharmacology, Astra Hässle AB, Mölndal, Sweden.

L.F. Gram, MD, Department of Clinical Pharmacology, Odense University, Denmark.

S.G. Grant, Department of Sports Science, University of Glasgow, Glasgow, Scotland.

J.D. Harry, BSc, MB BS, PhD, FFPM, Director, Drug Investigation and Clinical Research, Upjohn Ltd, Crawley, England.

J.G. McVie, BSc, MD, FRCPE, Director, Scientific Department, Cancer Research Campaign, London, England.

W.S. Nimmo, BSc, MD, FRCP, FFARCS, FFARACS, Inveresk Clinical Research, Edinburgh; Fellow in Anaesthesia, University of Edinburgh, Edinburgh, Scotland.

D.B. Northridge, MBChB, MRCP, Department of Cardiology, Western Infirmary, Glasgow, Scotland.

A. Petroccione, MD, Research and Development, Farmitalia Carlo Elba, Milano, Italy.

A. Pidgen, BSc, Hoechst Pharmaceuticals, Milton Keynes, England.

J. Posner, BSc, PhD, MBBS, MRCP, Department of Clinical Pharmacology, Wellcome Research Laboratories, Beckenham, Kent, England.

C. Praga, MD, Research and Development, Farmitalia Carlo Erba, Milano, Italy.

B. Tiplady, BA, PhD, Astra Clinical Research Unit, Edinburgh, Scotland.

F. Trave, MD, Research and Development, Farmitalia Carlo Erba, Milano, Italy.

G.T. Tucker, BPharm, PhD, Department of Medicine and Pharmacology, University of Sheffield, Sheffield, England.

J. Urquhart, MD, Chief Scientist, APREX Corporation, Fremont, CA, USA; Visiting Professor of Pharmaco-epidemiology, University of Limburg, Maastricht, The Netherlands.

T.R. Weihrauch, MD, Department of Medicine and Development, Pharmaceutical Research Centre, Bayer AG, Wuppertal, Germany.

B. Whiting, MD, FRCP, Professor of Clinical Pharmacology, Department of Medicine and Therapeutics, University of Glasgow, Scotland.

P.J. Wyld, MBChB, FRCP, MRCPath, Inveresk Clinical Research, Edinburgh, Scotland.

L.J.F. Youlten, MB, BS, MFPM, PhD, Head, Clinical Pharmacology Compliance, Smith Kline Beecham, Epsom, Surrey, England.

1. Introduction: Clinical Measurement and its Interpretation in Drug Evaluation

G.T. Tucker

In its broadest context, clinical measurement in drug evaluation covers phases I–IV – from the first introduction into man (usually healthy man), through studies in special patient groups and formal clinical trials, to post-marketing surveys of adverse events. The intention of this volume is to focus primarily on the methods of measuring specific pharmacological and therapeutic end-points, and, to a lesser extent, on the conduct of formal clinical trials, where the objective is mainly to assess clinical success or failure and the counting of bodies.

The measurement of the response to a drug involves four dimensions – dose, concentration, effect and time. Pharmacokineticists have spent the last 20 years establishing adequate tools for describing the dose–concentration–time paradigm. However, the more difficult task of measuring drug effects in man, especially in disease and as a function of time (pharmacodynamics), has tended to receive less attention, despite its obvious importance in drug development, evaluation and registration. In the UK at least, this has not been helped by a slow decline in academic clinical pharmacology over the past few years, accelerated by the virtual lack of funding for any research that does not involve sequencing the next gene. Nevertheless, there are some significant impetuses which may offset these trends. These include the advent of increasingly sophisticated instrumentation for physiological monitoring and biochemical analysis (culminating in the development of workable biosensors?), the elaboration of combined pharmacokinetic–pharmacodynamic and population modelling techniques (powerful approaches to optimising dosage regimens), the development of sophisticated drug delivery systems, and, hopefully, an increasing investment by the pharmaceutical industry in devising an improved methodology for measuring human drug response, both in-house and in collaboration with academic units. Incorporating these developments into the framework of early clinical studies should have substantial scientific and economic benefits with respect to the selection of optimal doses for full-scale clinical trials.

The scheme shown in *Figure 1.1* illustrates the various components of drug response. While this book is concerned primarily with the pharmacodynamic phase, it remains essential to appreciate pharmacokinetics, particularly when explaining inter- and intra-individual variability in response. It is important at this level to be relating response to the correct sort of drug concentration. Thus, free, unbound concentrations are often more relevant than total plasma

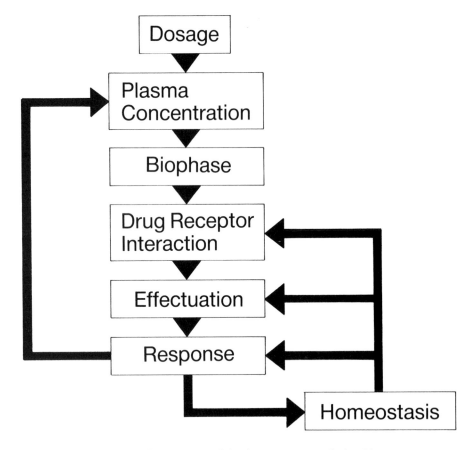

Figure 1.1. Components of the dose–response relationship.

or blood drug levels, and it is essential to define the active chemical moiety – whether it be parent compound, active metabolite or individual isomer. The site of blood sampling may also be a critical consideration when linking the time-course of drug concentration to the effect.

Within pharmacodynamics there are several layers to consider when interpreting the overall measure of effect, and it is vital to appreciate how dynamic the system is, involving time-delays and feedback readjustments. Thus, receptors are moving targets subject to homeostatic control by both up- and down-regulation. Post-receptor events (effectuation) often involve considerable changes in membrane permeability, formation of second messengers and biochemical reactions, all introducing potential time-delays. Finally, ultimate physiological or biochemical responses may feedback in the form of tolerance or amplification, either at the pharmacodynamic level or indirectly at a pharmacokinetic level, e.g., in the short term through cardiovascular adjustments affecting delivery of drug to and from sites of action or disposition, or in the longer term by phenomena such as enzyme induction. The control systems are complex and variable, thereby making considerable demands on how we approach making our measurements of effect and on how we interpret them.

It is important, therefore, to bear in mind some basic requirements for methods of measuring drug effect as we move through the contributions which constitute this volume.

Ideally, measurements should be appropriately **sensitive** – to changes in dose, concentration and pathophysiology when considering graded responses, and with respect to eliminating epiphenomena when considering quantum responses, such as adverse events. They should be **reproducible** within a subject and between investigators; **robust** in terms of ease of performance and susceptibility to external influences; **clinically relevant**; and **acceptable** both ethically and scientifically. Finally, and particularly important from a regulatory aspect, methods must, whenever possible, be **validated** with respect to accuracy using standard compounds and protocols.

2. Mortality in the Evaluation of Cardiovascular Drugs

R.W.F. Campbell

Introduction

Cardiovascular disease can cause a variety of symptoms and varying degrees of effort limitation. More seriously, many forms of cardiovascular disease can kill. While therapeutic interventions to prevent or modify cardiovascular disease may offer improved symptoms, increasing emphasis is being placed on developing treatments which will save life. Surgery and implantable electronic devices are important treatments which offer improved prognosis in selected situations, but drug therapy to reduce mortality has the advantages of its ease of implementation, relatively low cost, patient acceptability and flexibility for an individual approach.

Measuring mortality as an indicator of drug performance has many attractions. The diagnosis of death is objective and is not controversial. Mortality as an endpoint for drug evaluation, however, has important limitations. Patients may die by a different mechanism from that for which the protective therapy was designed. For instance, patients might receive an antiarrhythmic drug to prevent death by ventricular fibrillation. Even if effective for this purpose, the drug would not be expected to save the lives of patients who die of asystole. Mortality in survivors of myocardial infarction may result from several causes, of which arrhythmias and new ischaemia are but two. Thus, death is the final common result of varied pathological events. Different approaches are almost certainly necessary to deal with different mechanisms of death.

An approach to this problem in clinical studies has been to categorise death by mechanism or by time descriptors. Thus, arrhythmic death, death resulting from electromechanical dissociation, non-cardiac death, instantaneous death and sudden death are common endpoints in mortality studies. On casual examination, these categories would seem a reasonable approach but, in practice, categorising death is extremely difficult. All too often, death has been unwitnessed and categorisation must be by inference alone. Worse, there is little standardisation in the use of death categories. For instance, sudden death[10] in some studies has included only those patients who die within an hour of the onset of new symptoms, In other studies, the term implies instantaneous death, while in yet others, unwitnessed death in a patient who has been apparently stable within the last 24 hours might be included. It is easy to be critical of mortality studies, but it is extremely rare to have patients under such close surveillance that their true mode of death can be established. A compromise approach is essential, but its limitations must not be overlooked.

Selected Cardiovascular Drug Interventions that have Reduced Mortality

Many cardiovascular drugs are prescribed and investigated for reducing mortality, but only a few have been proved to offer this benefit. In some circumstances a drug may earn a reputation for mortality benefit on the basis of uncontrolled observations.

Beta-Blockers and Myocardial Infarction

In well-designed, randomised, double-blind studies, beta-blockers have improved the prognosis for survivors of myocardial infarction.[2,7,16] Overall, a 25% reduction in one-year mortality is obtained. The therapy is well tolerated by patients and important adverse effects are rare. Such has been the consistency of these trials that the medical community has interpreted the mortality benefit as a class effect.

In many countries, mortality benefits are being sought using beta-blockers which have not been the subject of controlled trials. New beta-blockers are often assumed, rightly or wrongly, to offer similar mortality benefits. Proving that they do, however, would be almost impossible as a placebo-controlled study of such patients would now be considered unethical.

Despite considerable research, the mechanism by which beta-blockers improve prognosis remains uncertain. The two leading theories are that the effects are either anti-ischaemic or antiarrhythmic. Establishing the protective mechanism is not of mere academic significance. That 75% of post-infarction mortality is not influenced by these agents would prompt a search for additional treatment which, depending upon the mechanism of beta-blocker protection, might be anti-ischaemic or antiarrhythmic.

Thrombolytic Therapy and Acute Phase Myocardial Infarction

Several well-controlled studies have established the beneficial mortality effects of thrombolytic therapy in acute phase myocardial infarction.[1,6,9] Benefits accrue to a wide range of patients, including (it would seem) those seen late after the onset of symptoms.[9] There is a suggestion from these studies that cardiac rupture may be more frequent in the first 24 hours of thrombolytic therapy[9], but this detrimental effect is obscured by the subsequent benefits. Thus, there is an overall gain, but at the possible expense of increased mortality in a small subgroup. In one acute intravenous beta-blocking study, cardiac rupture appeared to be reduced in those selected at random to receive atenolol.[8] It is tempting to suggest that a beta-blocker should be co-administered with thrombolytic therapy, but this would be an extrapolation from two different study populations. A formal study, which would be a considerable undertaking, would be necessary to ensure that the appropriate benefits are present with the combination of these drugs and that there is no unforeseen adverse interaction.

Beta-Blockers in the Congenital Long QT Syndromes

Mortality from sudden arrhythmic death is a serious and not uncommon complication of the congenital long QT syndromes. Meticulously collected patient data in an International Registry suggest that the prognosis is best for those patients treated with beta-adrenoreceptor blocking drugs and/or stellate ganglionectomy.[19] This treatment strategy has never been tested formally in a randomized study, but the observational data are so persuasive as to discourage such an investigation. This situation has the major disadvantage that new and potentially better therapies are unlikely to be tested in this population.

Vasodilatators and ACE Inhibitors in Severe Heart Failure

Heart failure carries a very grave prognosis. Death may be the result of an inexorable decline in cardiac mechanical performance or may be sudden and presumptively arrhythmic.[17] Until recently, no drug intervention had been shown to improve prognosis. Digoxin, diuretics, inotropic agents and antiarrhythmic drugs have all produced disappointing results, although they may offer symptomatic benefit. Vasodilator therapy, by contrast, does reduce mortality. The effect was first observed with the combination of isosorbide dinitrate and hydrallazine in the V-HeFT study[4], but was more strikingly revealed by enalapril in the CONSENSUS investigation.[5] This latter result was obtained in severe heart failure patients and it appears that the benefit arose from a reduction in mechanical death rather than in sudden death. It is easy to question the reliability of this observation, given the difficulty of defining and establishing that death was sudden and unexpected in a patient with severe heart failure. The mortality benefit is very important, but there are problems of interpretation. Can the effect be extrapolated to patients with lesser degrees of failure? Is the effect confined to enalapril or will other angiotensin converting enzyme (ACE) inhibitors offer the same benefit?

Selected Cardiovascular Drug Studies that have Increased Mortality

It is naive to believe that drugs can bring only good. Powerful drugs which may save lives also have the capacity to kill. In clinical practice, it would be unethical to test this effect; trials are usually designed on the premise that there will be benefit and are conducted to establish the risk of adverse effects in obtaining that benefit. A mortality study involving a drug would seem to involve a straightforward analysis, but an overall mortality result which does not examine cause of death may obscure groups of patients who are seriously disadvantaged by the therapy. An example would be that previously mentioned, in which cardiac rupture appeared increased in a thrombolytic trial in acute phase myocardial infarction.[9]

The problem can be illustrated by a hypothetical clinical condition which has a 10% one-year mortality. A useful drug intervention might reduce the annual mortality by 50%, such that only five patients in every 100 would die each year. But this same result might be seen with a drug intervention which saved the lives of eight patients who would otherwise have died, but which killed three patients who were not previously at risk. The net outcome of this scenario is that, to the casual observer, mortality is still reduced by 50%, but it has been achieved at a significant detriment to a small group of patients. Establishing whether such detrimental effects do occur in patient subsets is extremely difficult, but should be an important part of mortality studies.

In a few randomised controlled studies, either overall mortality was increased by the drug under investigation or a specific subgroup of patients suffered an unexpectedly high death rate.

Lidoflazine for Maintaining Sinus Rhythm

In a remarkable and disturbing study, lidoflazine was compared with quinidine in the maintenance of sinus rhythm after cardioversion for atrial fibrillation.[11] Quinidine and lidoflazine proved equally efficient at maintaining sinus rhythm, but a 27% mortality rate in patients receiving lidoflazine was unexpected and was sufficient to terminate the study.

Cardiac Arrhythmia Suppression Trial

Few studies have attained the notoriety of the Cardiac Arrhythmia Suppression Trial (CAST).[3] This investigation sought to establish whether suppression of ventricular ectopic beats in post-infarct survivors would be associated with an improvement in prognosis. Similar but smaller studies using a variety of antiarrhythmic agents had given little encouragement for this hypothesis, but many were flawed in their design and few examined the arrhythmias and antiarrhythmic drug effects in detail.[13] In CAST, the susceptibility of ventricular ectopic beats was established before randomisation. In this study, investigations of the effects of encainide and flecainide were terminated prematurely by a statistically significant excess mortality in those patients receiving active therapy. The mechanism of death has not been established adequately, but lethal arrhythmogenesis is a strong possibility. Modern day safety monitoring picked up the problem early and prevented more patients being put at risk. The result was important both scientifically (as it improved understanding of post-infarction risk) and clinically (as encainide and flecainide are now contraindicated for the purpose of reducing post-infarction mortality by ventricular ectopic beat suppression). The result has also caused a serious loss of confidence in these agents, which underscores the care with which mortality in drug trials must be interpreted. For a time, encainide and flecainide were under threat of withdrawal from clinical usage, despite the established fact that they are important and useful drugs for the treatment of reciprocating tachycardias and symptomatic ventricular arrhythmias. Inappropriate use post-infarction, as revealed by the increased mortality, was in this case wrongly extrapolated to other situations. Fortunately, prescribing guidelines were changed and these agents remain available for appropriate indications.

Clofibrate for Primary Prevention of Ischaemic Heart Disease (IHD)

In a well-designed, prospective randomised study, the primary protective effects of clofibrate were examined over a period of 208,000 man years.[18] Cardiovascular mortality was expected to be reduced. In the event, non-fatal myocardial infarction was significantly lowered, but both total mortality and non-IHD mortality were significantly increased. No clear explanation for this finding has been established, but this study, more than any other, has highlighted the need for remarkably safe therapy which is to be used as a primary preventative.

Selected Drug Intervention with no Mortality Effects

Many controlled studies using cardiovascular drugs have been undertaken with the intention of reducing mortality but have failed to show an effect. Poor study design, inadequate patient numbers, drug inefficacy, under-dosing, patient intolerance and a host of other technical factors are likely explanations. Although disappointing, these studies are important for our further understanding of the disease process. This is particularly the case when interventions may have improved symptoms, but not influenced mortality.

Management of hypertension can be justified on the basis of reducing fatal and non-fatal strokes, and this mortality benefit is offered by a variety of hypotensive agents.[14,15,20] Of great concern is the fact that there is no convincing evidence of cardiovascular mortality having been influenced by hypotensive drugs, despite their adequate effects on blood pressure. In heart failure management there is no evidence that diuretic therapy improves prognosis, yet these agents have important symptomatic benefits. Similarly, there is no evidence that the medical management of angina pectoris improves prognosis, although aspirin therapy has mortality benefits in patients with unstable angina.[12]

Mortality as a Clinical Measure

Prolonging life is an important clinical goal in cardiology. Surgery and electronic devices have a very important role for this purpose, but drugs, if effective, would have many advantages. New drugs which can modify mortality are needed. They will be developed and will need to be tested. Adequate evaluation necessitates detailed knowledge of the natural history of the condition. If given too late in the course of cardiovascular disease, a drug may stand no chance of offering benefit, even though it would prove beneficial for patients less severely compromised. Natural history information is sadly lacking. Long-term observational studies are demanding and have been relatively neglected in recent years. Placebo groups in large studies are another source of 'natural' history information, but the strict inclusion criteria and the often 'unnatural' management strategies imposed by such trials reduce the general applicability of the observations.

It is unrealistic to expect any single agent to ameliorate all mechanisms of death. *Total* mortality is and must remain the single most important result of a survival study, but drug actions may be highly selective. Concealed within statistically unchanged total mortality there may be patient subsets who either benefit or are disadvantaged. The fate of such patients is important, but this must not be interpreted as a primary result of the trial. To be seen as such, this subgroup would need to have been predefined and patients belonging to it to have been randomised appropriately.

References

[1] AIMS Trial Study Group. Long-term effects of intravenous anistreplase in acute myocardial infarction: final report of the AIMS Study. *Lancet*, **335**, 427–31, 1990.

[2] Beta Blocker Heart Attack Trial Research Group. A randomised trial of propranolol in patients with acute myocardial infarction. I: Mortality results. *JAMA*, **247**, 1707–14, 1982.

[3] Cardiac Arrhythmia Suppression Trial (CAST) Investigators. Preliminary report: effect of encainide and flecainide on mortality in a randomised trial of arrhythmia suppression after myocardial infarction. *N. Engl. J. Med.*, **321**, 406–12, 1989.

[4] Cohn, J.N., Archibald, D.G., Ziesche, S., Franciosa, J.A., Harston, W.E., Tristani, F.E., Dunkman, W.B., Jacobs, W., Francis, G.S., *et al.* Effect of vasodilator therapy on mortality in chronic congestive heart failure. Results of a Veterans Administration Cooperative study. *N. Engl. J. Med.*, **314**, 1547–52, 1986.

[5] CONSENSUS Trial Study Group. Effects of enalapril on mortality in severe congestive heart failure: results of the co-operative North Scandinavian Enalapril Survival Study (CONSENSUS). *N. Engl. J. Med.*, **316**, 1429–35, 1987.

[6] Gruppo Italiano per lo studio della streptochinasi nell infarto miocardico (GISSI). Long-term effects of intravenous thrombolysis in acute myocardial infarction: a final report of the GISSI study. *Lancet*, **2**, 871–4, 1987.

[7] Hjalmarson, A., Herlitz, J., and Holmberg, S. The Goteborg Metoprolol Trial: effects on mortality and morbidity in acute myocardial infarction. *Circulation*, **67** (Suppl I), 26–32, 1983.

[8] ISIS-1 Collaborative Group. Mechanism for the early mortality reduction produced by B-blockade started early in AMI. *Lancet*, **2** (8605), 292, 1988.

[9] ISIS-2 (Second International Study of Infarct Survival Collaborative Group). Randomised trial of intravenous streptokinase, oral aspirin, both, or neither among 17,187 cases of suspected acute myocardial infarction. *Lancet*, **2**, 349–60, 1988.

[10] Julian, D.G. and Campbell, R.W.F. Sudden death. In *Scientific Foundations of Cardiology*, Sleight, P., Vann Jones, J. (eds), William Heinemann Medical Books Ltd, London, pp. 220–4, 1983.

[11] Kennelly, B.M. Comparison of lidoflazine and quinidine in prophylactic treatment of arrhythmias. *Br. Heart J.*, **39**, 540–6, 1977.

[12] Lewis, H.D., David, J.W., Archibald, D.G., Heinke, W.E., Smitherman, P.C., Doherty, G.E., Schnaper, H.W., Le Winter, M.M., Linares, E., *et al.* Protective effects of aspirin against acute myocardial infarction and death in men with unstable angina. Results of a Veterans Administration Cooperative Study. *N. Engl. J. Med.*, **309**, 396–403, 1983.

[13] May, G.S., Eberlein, K.A., Furberg, C.D., Passamani, E.R., and DeMets, D.L. Secondary prevention after myocardial infarction: A review of long-term trials. *Prog. Cardiovasc. Dis.*, **24**, 331–52, 1982.

[14] Management Committee of the Australian Therapeutic Trial in Mild Hypertension. A report. *Lancet*, **i**, 1261–7, 1980.

[15] Medical Research Council Working Party. MRC trial of treatment of mild hypertension: principal results. *Br. Med. J.*, **291**, 97–104, 1985.

[16] Norwegian Multicenter Study Group. Timolol-induced reduction in mortality and reinfarction in patients surviving acute myocardial infarction. *N. Engl. J. Med.*, **304**, 801–807, 1981.

[17] Packer, M. Sudden unexpected death in patients with congestive heart failure: a second frontier. *Circulation*, **72**, 681–5, 1985.

[18] Report of the Committee of Principal Investigators. WHO Cooperative trial on primary prevention of ischaemic heart disease with clofibrate to lower serum cholesterol: final mortality follow-up. *Lancet*, **ii**, 600–4, 1984.

[19] Schwartz, P.J. The idiopathic long QT syndrome. The need for a prospective registry. *Eur. Heart J.*, **4**, 529–31, 1983.

[20] Veterans Administration Cooperative Study Group on Antihypertensive Agents. Effects of treatment on morbidity in hypertension: results in patients with diastolic blood pressures averaging 115 through 129 mmHg. *J. Am. Med. Assoc.*, **202**, 1029–34, 1967.

—

3. Exercise Testing in the Clinical Pharmacology of Heart Failure

H.J. Dargie, D.B. Northridge and S.G. Grant

Introduction

Heart failure is a clinical syndrome that may result from many causes, both cardiac and extra-cardiac. Thus, disease affecting the pericardium, endocardium, myocardium or the valves may so impair cardiac function that the heart cannot distribute sufficient oxygen for the metabolic needs of the body. In clinical trials of new drugs for combating heart failure, it is of crucial importance to define the population to be studied in terms of the question being asked. Thus, if it is important to demonstrate an improvement in effort capacity, the group selected should display decreased effort capacity. Moreover, because patients with diastolic failure may respond differently to a vasodilator than do those with systolic failure, it is important to include only patients with similar pathology. In most studies, a decreased left ventricular ejection fraction is the most reliable indicator of impaired systolic function.

Since heart failure has so many causes, in any investigation of drug action it is essential to diagnose the underlying cause. In clinical practice today, this is usually accomplished easily with a combination of the clinical features, the ECG and the echocardiogram; cardiac catheterisation and/or myocardial biopsy may also be required in some cases. In developed countries, by far the commonest cause of heart failure is myocardial failure resulting from coronary artery disease or dilated cardiomyopathy, which lead to impaired contractility (systolic failure). Increasingly recognised, but still less common, is a group of diseases often characterised by hypertrophy, where the principal abnormality is impaired relaxation (diastolic failure).[7]

In the assessment of the clinical pharmacology of a new drug to be used to treat heart failure, many standard invasive and non-invasive cardiological tests may be employed. Acute haemodynamic studies help by confirming the general classification of drug type, i.e., vasodilator or inotrope. Symptom assessments by means of direct questioning or some form of self-perception scoring, such as the visual analogue or Likert scales, have proved reliable, while quality-of-life questionnaires are a more recent approach.[5,6] Obviously mortality is an important end point (see page 9).

At the present time, improvement of exercise capacity is seen by drug regulatory authorities as a key factor in assessing new drug applications. In this chapter, therefore, we review the basic considerations in exercise testing and propose a novel approach that would, to a great extent, ease the problem of multicentre exercise testing.

The Problem

The fundamental problem is not just that some investigators, especially in the USA and UK, use treadmills while others, particularly in continental Europe, use bicycles for exercise testing, but also that different protocols may be used within either mode of exercise, most of which are eponymous rather than descriptive. The exercise capacity recorded at the end of the test is often referred to in terms of the workload in watts for a bicycle test and in minutes for the treadmill.

The Physiological Basis of Exercise Testing[14]

The currency of exercise is oxygen and its consumption per kilogram of body weight during exercise is closely related to the physiological sequelae of exercise, including tachycardia and rise in arterial pressure. Oxygen uptake ($\dot{V}O_2$) is described most correctly in ml/kg/min. At rest the $\dot{V}O_2$ is approximately 3.5 ml/kg/min, which is often referred to as 1 metabolic equivalent (1 MET).[1]

It is apparent from *Figure 3.1* that the measured energy costs expressed as $\dot{V}O_2$ in ml/kg/min during bicycle exercise vary inversely with body weight while, during treadmill exercise, they are similar for all subjects at the same stage of exercise. Thus, to reach a $\dot{V}O_2$ of 25 ml/kg/min (approx. 7 MET) would take:

- 5 min for a 60 kg person starting at 20 W and increasing by 20 W/min to 100 W.

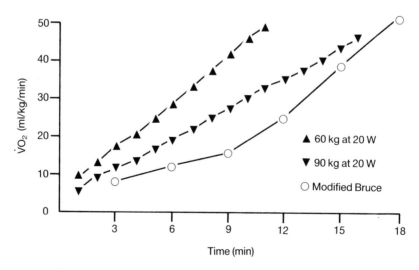

Figure 3.1. Energy requirements of currently used exercise tests.

- 8 min (>60% longer) for a 90 kg person on a bicycle.
- 12 min for either subject on a modified Bruce treadmill protocol.

The duration of an exercise test is important, but so too is how hard the exercise feels to the individual. It seems self-evident that, in attempting to achieve comparability within a multicentre study, the exercise testing experience should be as similar as possible for each patient. Moreover, analysis of the data would be greatly facilitated by the range of exercise times being influenced only by patient factors, such as baseline ability and change in clinical status, rather than also by differences in exercise testing protocol.

Which Test?

No exercise protocol is satisfactory for all populations; a test used in a hospital setting is, for example, of little value for elite athletes. Moreover, patients exhibit a broad spectrum of exercise capacity and this creates difficulty in devising a test that is appropriate for all subjects. However, no matter the population, an aerobic test should progress from initial workloads which can be accomplished easily, to workloads which increase gradually until the subject reaches his maximum capacity.[8]

The optimum duration of an aerobic test should be 10–20 min[8], although some researchers have concluded that work-rate increments should be selected to bring most subjects to maximum in 10 ±2 min.[4] Clearly it is very difficult to realise these recommendations in untried subjects. For instance, when the patients cover a wide range of capabilities, the investigator is faced with a dilemma when testing: a test which starts with very low energy costs to accommodate subjects with a poor exercise capacity will result in a very long test for better performers. However, long tests may produce unrepresentative values as subjects may become bored, experience discomfort or lack commitment for a sustained effort. Conversely, short duration tests with large energy cost increments may limit the attainment of a true maximum, as the subject will experience difficulty in coping with large energy cost increases between stages.

Bicycle or Treadmill?

Bicycles and treadmills are both commonly used to assess aerobic capability. The bicycle has several advantages over the treadmill.[9] The subject's upper body is in a stable position which facilitates the recording of the ECG, measurement of arterial pressure and blood sampling. In addition, there is less variation in energy costs between subjects on the bicycle compared with those on the treadmill.[2] However, maximum oxygen uptake has been consistently reported to be approximately 8% lower on a bicycle than on a treadmill.[10] One contributory factor may be localised fatigue of the quadriceps during bicycle testing. When treadmill protocols incorporate increases in speed and changes in gradient at the same stage, subjects can become unsettled. Furthermore, it has been demonstrated that the test duration can be greatly increased if the subject holds the handrails during a treadmill test.[13]

It is possible to calculate the approximate rates of energy expenditure required to perform exercise workloads on treadmills and bicycle ergometers.

As the body weight is supported by the saddle of the bicycle, the oxygen cost per kilogram of body weight is less for heavier subjects. Despite this, the designs of bicycle protocols usually do not take body weight into consideration.

Although several treadmill exercise tests are very popular, most are open to criticism. For example, the Bruce test has abrupt increases in workload between stages, while the Balke and Naughton tests are too long for fit subjects.[12] Furthermore, the gradient of some tests can produce low back pain and/or calf pain.

Can the same Protocol be Applied to Bicycle and Treadmill?

It can be seen, from *Figure 3.1*, that the energy costs per unit time of bicycle and treadmill protocols in current use are grossly dissimilar.

The relative energy costs are theoretically identical for all treadmill exercise, though there will be some variability between subjects related to the efficiency of walking and whether the handrail is held or not. Taking the Bruce protocol as an example, we have constructed bicycle protocols for subjects of varying weight, to mirror the energy costs predicted from Bruce's regression equation in the initial validation of his test.[3] Thus each subject has an individualised bicycle protocol and we measure the oxygen uptake of all subjects during that bicycle test and during the Bruce protocol. These results are shown in *Table 3.1*. The actual energy costs for both modes of exercise were very similar, thus demonstrating that it is possible to reproduce the relative energy costs of one mode of exercise while using the other.

There were, however, a number of differences, including a slightly but significantly greater double product on bicycle exercise, together with a greater sense of leg fatigue.

Table 3.1. Mean energy cost (ml/kg/min) of bicycle and treadmill tests.

	Bruce regression equation	*Bicycle test*	*Treadmill test*
Stage 1	17.0	17.4 (16.0, 18.8)	14.6 (13.5, 15.7*)
Stage 2	26.0	24.7 (23.5, 25.8*)	21.0 (19.5, 22.6*)
Stage 3	35.0	32.2 (31.0, 35.7)	31.0 (28.9, 33.1*)
Stage 4	44.0	41.5 (39.0, 44.0)	43.8 (40.2, 47.3)

* Significantly different from the Bruce equation.

Can We do Better than the Bruce Protocol?

The prospect of a protocol which can be applied to a wide range of subjects is appealing. Furthermore, the possibility of a protocol which has approximately the same energy cost increases for both the bicycle and the treadmill would be of value in comparing subjects tested in either mode. Such a test should start at a low energy cost and should increase exponentially, thus catering for very low fitness levels, while also accommodating fitter subjects. We have devised a new exercise test which can be applied to a wide range of cardiac patients.[11]

Standardised Exponential Exercise Protocol (the STEEP Test)

Initially, a treadmill protocol was designed with one minute stages, beginning with a low workload (2 MET) and increasing by 15%/min for 15 min (STEEP test) [*Table 3.2*]. This produced an exponential rise in workloads, with small increases initially and larger rises (maximum of 1.4 MET/min) at the end of the test. The STEEP test was validated in 20 normal subjects, all of whom completed the 15 min protocol. The mean (SD) oxygen consumption was 9.0 (1.7) ml/min/kg during the first stage of the test, and rose exponentially to 40.4(5.1) ml/min/kg during the final stage (*Figure 3.2*).

Table 3.2. STEEP treadmill protocol.

	Stage (min)														
	1	2	3	4	5	6	7	8	9	10	11	12	13	14	15
Speed (m.p.h.)	1.5	2.0	2.0	2.0	2.5	2.5	2.5	3.0	3.0	3.0	3.5	3.5	3.5	4.2	5.0
Speed (km/h)	2.4	3.2	3.2	3.2	4.0	4.0	4.0	4.8	4.8	4.8	5.6	5.6	5.6	6.7	8.0
Elevation (%)	0	0	1.5	3	3	5	7	7	9	11	11	13	16	16	16

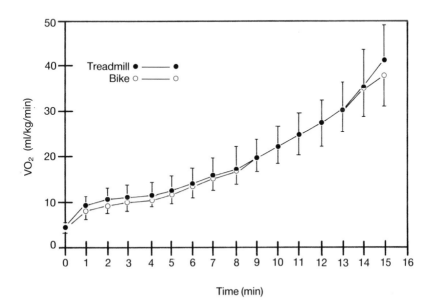

Figure 3.2. Energy requirements of the STEEP exercise protocol.

With the small energy cost increases in the early stage of the test, the measured oxygen cost mirrored the estimated energy cost. As expected, the larger energy cost increments during the latter stages resulted in a slightly lower measured oxygen consumption than the predicted values. The relatively small energy cost increments resulted in a 'comfortable' test for all subjects. Subjects who had experienced other tests remarked on this aspect, compared with the abrupt stage increases of the Bruce protocol.

In addition, the STEEP protocol has been used in patients with varying severity of heart failure. The exercise times of ten patients varied from 4.7 min to 10.6 min and peak oxygen consumption ranged from 12.5 ml/min/ kg to 20.4 ml/min/kg. All patients found the test simple to perform (*Figure 3.3*).

We have calculated the same energy cost increments for bicycle exercise (*Table 3.3*), and preliminary work has been carried out to compare the STEEP protocol on a bicycle and a treadmill (*Figure 3.2*). These tests and our previous ones using the Bruce protocol show that it is possible to prescribe an exercise test on a bicycle and a treadmill with very similar energy costs. Thus, a comparison between different modes of testing can be made. However, it should be noted that this and other studies have shown that the perceived level of leg fatigue is higher on a bicycle, while numerous studies indicate that maximum oxygen uptake is lower on a bicycle. It is anticipated, therefore, that maximum tests with a patient population will always produce a slightly shorter test duration on a bicycle as compared with a treadmill.

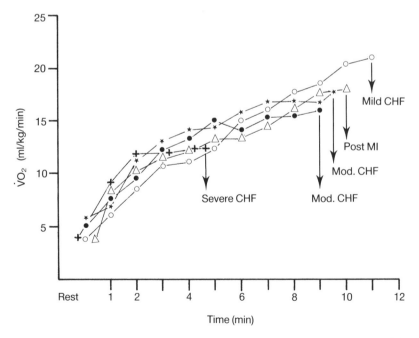

Figure 3.3. Energy requirements of the STEEP protocol in patients with heart failure (CHF, cardiac heart failure; MI, myocardial infarction).

Table 3.3. STEEP bicycle protocol showing the workload for each of the 15 stages of the protocol as determined by the subject's body weight (kg).

Weight (kg)	Stage														
	1	2	3	4	5	6	7	8	9	10	11	12	13	14	15
50	15	20	25	30	40	50	60	70	85	95	110	125	145	170	185
55	15	20	30	35	45	55	65	80	95	105	125	140	160	185	205
60	15	25	30	40	45	60	70	85	100	115	135	150	175	200	225
65	20	25	35	40	50	65	80	90	110	125	145	165	190	220	240
70	20	25	35	45	55	70	85	100	120	135	155	175	205	235	260
75	20	30	40	45	60	75	90	105	125	145	170	190	220	250	280
80	25	30	40	50	65	80	95	115	135	155	180	200	235	270	295
85	25	35	45	55	65	85	100	120	145	165	190	215	250	285	315
90	25	35	45	55	70	90	105	130	150	175	200	225	265	300	335
95	25	35	50	60	75	95	115	135	160	180	215	240	280	320	350
100	30	40	50	65	80	100	120	140	170	190	225	250	295	335	370

Nonetheless, the STEEP protocol has the advantage that it can be applied to both bicycle and treadmill. Furthermore, the more physiological energy cost increments have resulted in a test duration which is more acceptable, when applied to a wide-ranging population, than those of other stress tests. Thus, the STEEP protocol allows for comparison between different modes of test and can be applied to a wide range of patients.

The Exercise Testing Procedure

In clinical pharmacology especially, but also in clinical practice, there should be as much standardisation as can be achieved. If possible, all testing centres should have similar equipment which facilitates calibration (on each day that study is performed) and minimises variability resulting from factors such as saddle discomfort and cadence (rate of pedalling). Laboratory temperature should be maintained at 18–22°C. Clothing should be conducive to performing the test; shorts are best, as are trainers or flat rubber-soled shoes.

Whenever possible, the same technician or doctor should test the patient each time at approximately the same time of day and the same time after ingestion of the trial drug. Three hours post-prandial and drug ingestion could be adopted.

As far as drugs are concerned, cigarette smoking should be prohibited (especially with dihydropyridines), and coffee and tea should be avoided during the two hours before the test. No alcohol should be permitted from 22.00 on the previous evening. Glyceryl trinitrate should not be taken for at least one hour before testing.

For bicycle exercise, the subject should be weighed (to the nearest kilogram) in shorts and shirt with no shoes. Selection of the appropriate workload is made by referring to *Table 3.3*.

A one-minute period of exercise at the initial workload serves as a warm-up and establishes the correct leg length (i.e., leg almost straight when pedal is , fully down) and that the patient is capable of sustaining a cadence of 60 revs/min. Handlebars should be held lightly. Toe clips (which are advantageous for patients unfamiliar with bicycle exercise and do not impede those who are) should be standard.

The test procedure should be explained to the patients who should be told that there will be a one-minute warm-up to allow familiarisation with the apparatus. During this period, it should be established that the patient is comfortable and can maintain the appropriate cadence. Thereafter the patient stops pedalling. It is then explained that the test will become progressively harder every minute, and that when the patient wishes to stop, he should signal (thumbs down). Immediately the workload will be reduced. The patient should continue to pedal at a low workload to facilitate recovery. It should be stressed that he should attempt to attain the longest duration possible during the incremental test.

The investigator should gently encourage the patient as appropriate at each stage of the test, thereby generating confidence and rapport. The degree of encouragement should be similar for all patients. The decision to terminate a test may be taken by:

- The investigator, when some predetermined end point has been reached.
- The patient, when he is certain that he wishes to stop.
- Both the patient and the doctor, usually as a result of dialogue between them. This can never be standardised completely, but no undue encouragement should be given, especially when symptoms such as chest pain have appeared. However, if the doctor considers all is well, he should say so.

To prevent venous pooling, the patient should be asked to continue walking or pedalling at the initial (lowest) workload for 2 min, at zero load for a further 2 min, and to rest for a final 2 min.

Arterial pressure should be measured using a mercury sphygmomanometer at cuff height on an arm held loosely (i.e., not holding handlebars or handrail).

Conclusions

The increasing application of bicycle and treadmill exercise testing in an area of increasing regulation and demands for accuracy and reliability, such as the clinical pharmacology of heart failure, requires a reconsideration of objectives and protocol. It is only by greater standardisation and attention to detail that the exercise test will be elevated from its present status, as a universal clinical test where the 'noise' in the system may be so great that differentiation of subtle but important drug effects is often impossible.

References

[1] American College of Sports Medicine. Guidelines for exercise testing and prescription. 3rd edition. Lea & Febiger, Philadelphia, 1986.
[2] Astrand, P.O. and Rodahl, K. *Physiological bases of exercise. Textbook of*

Work Physiology. 3rd edition. McGraw-Hill Book Company, New York, St Louis, San Francisco, 1986.

[3] Bruce, R.A. Exercise testing of patients with coronary heart disease. Principles and normal standards for evaluation. *Annals of Clinical Research*, **3**, 323–32, 1971.

[4] Buchfuhrer, M.J., Hansen, J.E., Robinson, T.E., Sue, D.T., Wasserman, K., and Whipp, B.J. Optimising the exercise protocol for cardiopulmonary assessment. *Journal of Applied Physiology*, **55** (5), 1558–64, 1983.

[5] Cleland, J.G.F., Dargie, H.J., Ball, S.G., *et al*. Effects of enalapril in heart failure: a double blind study of effects on exercise performance, renal function, hormones and metabolic state. *Br. Heart J.*, **54**, 305–12, 1985.

[6] German and Austrian Xamoterol Study Group. Double blind placebo-controlled comparison of digoxin and xamoterol in chronic heart failure. *Lancet*, **ii**, 489, 1988.

[7] Hamilton, A., Naccarelli, G.V., Gray, I.L., *et al*. Congestive heart failure with normal systolic function. *Am. J. Cardiol.* **84**, 778, 1984.

[8] Lamb, D.R. *Physiology of Exercise. Responses and adaptations. Evaluation of cardiovascular function and aerobic endurance performance*. 2nd edition. MacMillan Publishing Company, New York; Collier MacMillan Publishers, London, pp. 173–90, 1984.

[9] McKirnan, M.D. and Froelicher, V.F. General principles of exercise testing. In *Exercise Testing and Exercise Prescription or Special Cases*, J.S. Skinner (ed), Lea & Febiger, Philadelphia, pp. 3–19, 1987.

[10] Miles, D.S., Critz, J.B., and Knowlton, R.G. Cardiovascular, metabolic and ventilatory responses of women to equivalent cycle ergometer and treadmill exercise. *Medicine and Science in Sports and Exercise*, **12** (1), 14–19, 1986.

[11] Northridge, D.B., Grant, S., Ford, I., *et al*. Novel exercise protocol suitable for use on a treadmill or a bicycle ergometer. *Br. Heart J.*, **64**, 313–6, 1990.

[12] Pollock, M.L., Wilmore, J.H., and Fox, S.M. *Exercise in Health and Disease*. W.B. Saunders Company, Philadelphia, 1984.

[13] Ragg, K.E., Murray, T.F., Karbonit, L.M., and Jump, D.A. Errors in predicting functional capacity from a treadmill exercise stress test. *Am. Heart J.* **100** (4), 581–3, 1989.

[14] Sheffield, L.T. Exercise stress testing in heart disease. In *Heart Disease*, Braunwald, E. (ed), W.B. Saunders, Philadelphia, pp. 223–41, 1988.

4. The Monitoring of Arterial Pressure

J.D. Harry

Introduction

The term 'arterial pressure' refers to the pressure of the blood in the arterial side of the circulation. The pressure is essential to life because upon it depends the passage of blood, with its constituents, to the various organs of the body. Its measurement in man has been possible for many years since the development of the occluding cuff techniques by various workers[34,19], including Korotkoff[21] who gave his name to the sounds which can be heard in an artery below a cuff as it is slowly reduced from above systolic pressure to below diastolic blood pressure. (Korotkoff 1st sound indicates systolic pressure, and IV or V diastolic pressure – see review by Raftery[32] for merits of IV and V to estimate the diastolic pressures.) The pressures in the cuff are measured via a mercury or aneroid manometer attached to the cuff. Such methods are the indirect methods of measuring arterial pressure in a human arm, referred to as sphygmomanometry cuff techniques (or osculatory techniques).

It has become clear that single casual arterial pressure measurements (as made in a practitioner's surgery) can be influenced by many factors. Thus analysis of repeated measurements over a period of time, as may be required to assess the effect of a drug on arterial pressure, may be very difficult.

Factors Affecting Measurements of Arterial Pressure

These can be divided essentially into two categories: those factors related to techniques and those related to biological variability of the arterial pressure in man.

The problems that can occur under the heading of 'faulty techniques' have been well reviewed by Petrie et al.[30], who give recommendations concerning the menisci of the mercury column in a mercury manometer, width of cuff, deflation rate in the cuff, etc. 'Digit' bias is a common source of error in measuring arterial pressure, e.g. 'to the closest 2 or 5 mmHg'. To assess the effect of a drug on arterial pressure over weeks or months, technical faults such as these need to be kept to a minimum. The use of the Hawksley Random Zero machine or the London School of Tropical Medicine and Hygiene Machine helps to minimise some of the errors.[32]

Biological variation of arterial pressure is now well recognised. Included is the basic circadian variation, whereby high values are recorded at midmorning and fall from that point throughout the day to reach the lowest values during sleep, before rising again close to waking.[25] Arterial pressure can also rise as a result of the 'alarm' or 'alerting' reaction induced in a subject by the fact of having his arterial pressure recorded.[24] Further factors, such as exercise, posture, smoking, etc., are all known to affect the measurements.[10]

The techniques which are now available to measure arterial pressure have been developed in an attempt to take into account such variability. This ensures that more reliable measurements can be made in an individual to assess the presence (or otherwise) of hypertension, and equally importantly to assess the effects of appropriate therapy. These same techniques are also used during clinical development to estimate the effects of new compounds on arterial pressure.

Methods Available to Measure Arterial Pressure

These can be divided into indirect and direct methods. The former rely upon the 'occlusion and detection' methods already discussed, essentially involving the brachial artery, while the latter employ a catheter inserted directly into an artery (normally the brachial or radial artery) and attached to a pressure transducer. Both types of method measure arterial pressure, but, while the indirect methods are intermittent, the direct ones are continuous, measuring beat-to-beat changes induced by the heart rhythm. These two sets of recordings therefore give different perspectives of the arterial pressure, and consequently the use of one or the other will depend upon the monitoring required during a particular investigation. The techniques of the various methods have been reported in numerous reviews over the years.[32,35] It is not intended to restate these technical details here, but rather to look at the advantages and disadvantages of the different methods for monitoring arterial pressure in the evaluation of new drugs.

Indirect Methods

The greatest advantage of the occluding cuff technique, used with a stethoscope to detect changes in sounds, lies in its familiarity to workers in the field of drug evaluation. The inherent faults within this system have been described earlier and can be overcome with the London School of Hygiene and Tropical Medicine and Hawksley Random Zero machines. However, the use of these machines does require careful training, and the readings can refer only to 'one-off' carefully controlled measurements in a laboratory or outpatient setting. Calibration and computational errors can still occur.[11,38] The machines can really only be used with the patient at rest and thus it is almost impossible to record arterial pressure in this way during exercise. Finally, the 'alerting reaction' and other biological variations in arterial pressure are not reduced by using these instruments.

Attempts to reduce some of the biological variations have been made by allowing patients to measure their own arterial pressure in their own homes[20], a technique that has been used to assess some antihypertensive agents.[6] Several assessments of arterial pressure recorded by patients themselves during the day do reflect pressures recorded by direct arterial catheterisation, although morning and evening pressures alone may not reflect the mean blood pressure recorded throughout the day.[15]

This method easily allows assessment of arterial pressure more frequently than do clinic measurements and some of the biological variations can be reduced, but it still has limitations. These are that patients need the ability and inclination to be trained in the technique, that knowledge of their own arterial pressures may influence the readings, and finally that little data on conditions other than those when at rest can be obtained, and that no data can be obtained at all at night.

Automated devices have been introduced to 'remove the observer' from the measurement of blood pressures and to control cuff deflation rates, etc. All depend upon the principal of arterial occlusion and the detection of changes in the artery, either by sounds (with a microphone, e.g. Remler apparatus) or by movement of the arterial wall (using ultrasound, e.g. Arteriosond, or oscillometry, e.g. Dinamap). The automated machines allow even greater possibilities for self-measurement of arterial pressure by patients at various times throughout the day. At present, there is a plethora of such devices available for use in diagnosing and treating patients for hypertension. However, although some of these devices have been validated properly[7,12,18], not all have been, and the very necessary validation of these techniques has come under the scrutiny of the British Hypertension Society. This society now recommends that manufacturers provide evidence of validation of their machines, using guidelines similar to those laid down by the Association for the Advancement of Medical Instrumentation[1], and that validation should be published in reputable journals. Despite these recommendations, evidence is growing that some of these automated devices, while acceptable for assessing standard arterial pressures, are not sufficient when a patient has been treated with drugs that change the arterial pressure acutely, e.g. isoprenaline. The results in *Figure 4.1* show that the Nippon–Colin machine (an oscillometric device) grossly underestimated the drop in diastolic pressure induced by intravenous isoprenaline in comparison with a standard sphygmomanometer and cuff (Accosan) in normal volunteers, a result also found with the Dinamap machine when compared with direct intra-arterial measurement.[2] This may be a problem only with oscillometric automated devices, but that remains to be determined.

This evidence points to the fact that each of these automated machines needs validation in the centre where it is to be used and for the investigation procedure to be followed.

Direct Methods

The direct monitoring of arterial pressure is possible, but it involves the insertion of a fine catheter into the brachial or radial artery. Systems should be available to prevent clotting (normally the catheter undergoes constant perfusion), to measure pressure (i.e. a miniaturised pressure transducer), and to record the pressures (i.e. a magnetic tape), in this way allowing the continuous recording of arterial pressure. Such systems have been available for some years[31] and have been validated.[20] Computer analyses are required to handle the massive amount of data that represents the arterial pressure

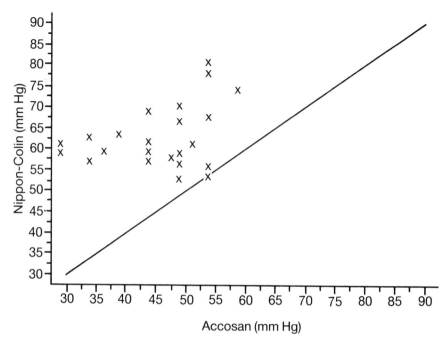

Figure 4.1. Diastolic pressures after isoprenaline administration measured by the Nippon–Colin machine and by the Accosan sphygmomanometer. Each point records the measurement of both machines at various infusion rates of isoprenaline (0, 1.0, 2 and 4 μgm/kg/min) from six volunteers; ——— = line of identity.

each time the heart beats. Most centres that use this technique plot mean hourly arterial pressures over a 24-hour period.[25] However, the method does allow estimates of variability of the arterial pressure to be made over a given time period, and this may be another way to monitor changes induced by drugs.

There can be no doubt that intra-arterial pressure recordings are the most accurate assessments of arterial pressure that can be made. Recording the pressure in the absence of an observer, the system is also ambulatory, which means that subjects' pressure during normal daily activity and sleep can be monitored accurately. Provided that the activity of patients remains relatively constant from day to day, the technique is reproducible to allow the effects of drugs to be monitored.[13]

Comparisons of 'direct' with 'indirect' methods have been made.[4,33] Overall the correlations are reasonable, with the indirect methods producing lower pressures for systolic pressures (about 3 mmHG) and higher diastolic pressures (16–17 mmHg for phase IV and 6–7 mmHg for V). However, the point made in both articles[4,33] was that these mean values did not reflect some of the larger differences which were seen at specific time points. Systolic pressure could be higher by as much as 18 mmHg or lower by 30 mmHg, and the diastolic (phase V) by +28 and −15 mmHg. These methods are assessing different measurements, with direct methods measuring continuous beat-to-beat changes in arterial pressure and the indirect methods measuring intermittent one-off measurements.

A non-invasive method, 'Finapres', is now available to measure beat-to-beat changes in arterial pressure. This measures the pressure in the finger (usually the index finger) using a 'volume clamp method'. Comparisons have been made between this method and direct pressure recordings from the radial or brachial arteries. The indirect method does appear to provide an accurate estimate of means and variability of arterial pressures in a group of subjects in a laboratory setting.[29] One possible problem with 'Finapres' may be the effects of local vasoconstriction on the measurements of arterial pressures, but one study suggests this criticism is unjustified.[8] Clearly, further evidence is required to determine whether 'Finapres' is a viable alternative to direct arterial pressure recordings, at least in a laboratory setting with the subject at rest.

Non-Invasive Ambulatory Monitoring of Arterial Pressure

The evidence obtained from the direct measurements of arterial pressure has allowed accurate monitoring of the effects of drugs on this pressure. However, it has the major disadvantage of being invasive with the inherent risk of catheterising an artery for a long period of time. This has resulted in the development of non-invasive ambulatory monitoring techniques in an attempt to obtain pressure monitoring in patients during their normal daily lives over a long period of time (up to 24 or 48 hours). A number of these devices are now available and some are listed in *Table 4.1*. All use the

Table 4.1. Some currently available non-invasive ambulatory arterial pressure monitoring devices.

Name of equipment	Method to detect blood pressure	Weight (kg)
Remler M-2000 (semi automatic)	Auscultatory	0.7
Spacelabs 90202	Oscillometric	0.6
Accutracker	Auscultatory	1.2
Pressurometer	Oscillometric	0.8

Table 4.2. Assessments required to validate a non-invasive automated ambulatory monitoring device.

1. Accuracy and reliability against a mercury manometer.
2. Accuracy in use on people against a standard Sphygmomanometer (preferably random zero) or inter-arterial blood pressure.
3. Acceptability to subjects.
4. Reproducibility (repeat whole day measurements before and after treatment with placebo for a period of time).
5. Sensitivity (estimate change that could be detected following treatment with placebo).

occlusion/detection technique with the pressure being recorded onto magnetic tape for subsequent replay from a decoding machine of some kind. As with the automated devices for measuring arterial pressure in the clinic or laboratory setting, these machines require validation before use. The type of information required from such a validation programme (*Table 4.2*) has been provided by Conway *et al.* at Oxford for their own ambulatory machine.[5] This type of excellent data should be provided for any ambulatory device and, as with static automated machines, recommendations for the information which should be provided are being considered by the British Hypertension Society.[28]

Non-invasive ambulatory monitoring of arterial pressure is not the same as direct ambulatory monitoring. The former gives intermittent measures of arterial pressure (usually at half-hour intervals throughout the day) and the latter gives continuous beat-to-beat changes.[27] Initially, it was possible to record arterial pressure only during the daytime with the non-invasive ambulatory techniques, because devices were not fully automated and were noisy, but now some machines are available which do not disturb the subjects during sleep. Thus, non-invasive ambulatory monitoring of arterial pressure can be used effectively to determine the effects of drugs on this pressure.[9,16] Furthermore, evidence is now accumulating to indicate that drugs which lower arterial pressure in the clinic setting may not do so when the effects are measured by ambulatory techniques. Thus nitrendipine effectively lowers arterial pressures in the clinic, but the effect is blunted on ambulatory measurements during work periods[37], perhaps because of increased sympathetic nervous activity which will not be affected by a calcium antagonist. To support this hypothesis, β-adrenoceptor blocking agents have been shown to reduce blood pressures measured using ambulatory techniques.[36] This type of evidence does now make it mandatory for new antihypertensive agents to be monitored with ambulatory techniques (direct or indirect).

Monitoring of Arterial Pressure during the Evaluation of New Drugs

The essential reasons for monitoring arterial pressure during the evaluation of new drugs are summarised in *Table 4.3*. Safety is an important issue for a putative drug and, should any new compound produce changes in arterial pressure, these need to be known. If these changes are of sufficient magnitude, the compound may be withdrawn from development. The use of ambulatory monitoring in this respect may be of immense value. If, during

Table 4.3. Reasons to monitor arterial pressure in the evaluation of new drugs.

1. Safety
2. Efficacy
3. Use of arterial pressure as a pharmacological model in man
4. Part of the assessment in studies of haemodynamics of a compound affecting the cardiovascular system

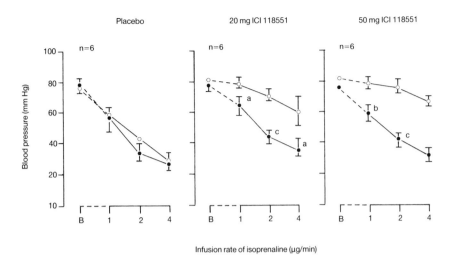

Figure 4.2. Effects of intravenous isoprenaline on the diastolic blood pressure in six normal volunteers before and after single oral doses of placebo or ICI 118551 (20 and 50 mg). Each point is mean value ± SEM; •——• before placebo or ICI 118551; ○——○ after placebo or ICI 118551; B = before infusing isoprenaline; $^a p<0.05$, $^b p<0.01$, $^c p<0.0001$ – comparing before and after placebo or drug.

the evaluation of a compound, reports are made that the compound is producing side-effects which could be attributed to postural hypotension, then this could easily be confirmed by ambulatory monitoring of the blood pressure.

Drugs that may act on the heart or the cardiovascular system may require haemodynamic assessments, usually by invasive techniques (e.g. antiarrhythmic agents, inotropic agents). These will always include a direct assessment of arterial pressure. Using the invasive haemodynamic approach, it may be possible to assess the mechanism of the change in arterial pressure should it occur.

The measurement of arterial pressure can be used as a model in humans to determine whether the pharmacology seen in animal models occurs in man. Changes in arterial pressure induced by isoprenaline can be used to demonstrate whether a β-adrenoceptor blocking agent is cardioselective in man. The fall in diastolic pressure induced by isoprenaline can be attenuated by the β_2-selective blocking agent ICI 118551, while the rise in systolic pressure cannot (*Figures 4.2* and *4.3*). Furthermore, the increase in systolic pressure induced by exercise is not attenuated by ICI 118551 (*Figure 4.4*). The conclusion drawn from these results is that the fall in diastolic pressure induced by isoprenaline is essentially dependent upon stimulation of β_2-adrenoceptors, while the changes in systolic pressure by isoprenaline and exercise are β_1 effects. With this knowledge, a putative β_1-selective agent can be tested for differential effects on these β_1- and β_2-dependent changes in arterial pressure.[17]

Arterial pressure is monitored to the greatest extent when a new antihypertensive agent is under evaluation. Initial studies can be performed in

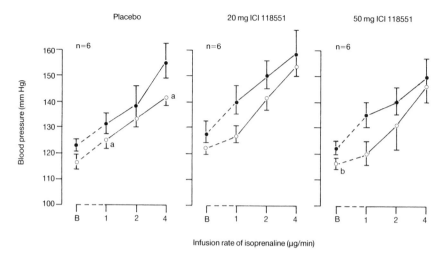

Figure 4.3. Effects of intravenous isoprenaline on the systolic blood pressure in six normal volunteers before and after single oral doses of placebo and of ICI 118551 (20 and 50 mg). Each point is mean value ± SEM; ●——● before placebo or ICI 118551; ○——○ after placebo or ICI 118551; B = before infusing isoprenaline; $^a p < 0.05$, $^b p < 0.01$ – comparing before and after placebo or drug.

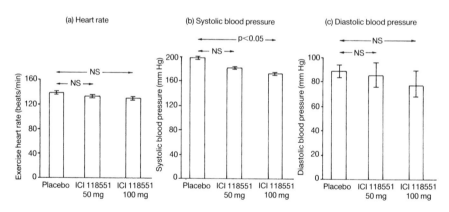

Figure 4.4. Effects of single oral doses of placebo and ICI 118551 (50 and 100 mg) on heart rate and arterial pressure responses to exercise. Each bar represents the mean ± SEM from six volunteers.

volunteers using standard sphygmomanometry techniques, whether these be automated or not, provided errors are reduced by careful attention to the details of measurements as suggested by Petre *et al.*[30] The results may provide some idea of efficacy and safety, in particular indicating a dose with which to proceed into Phase II studies in patients with hypertension. In these patients, the requirement to demonstrate efficacy should now be more strict than in the past. Efficacy should be shown in the clinic, in the home (with patients monitoring their own arterial pressure) and also in ambulatory states. From these studies should come evidence of the effect of the drug in lying, standing, work, exercise and sleeping situations. The ideal method for these studies should be direct invasive ambulatory monitoring for at least 24 hours. Even with invasive methods, attempts should be made to 'standardise' activities in the patient studied on different days, especially if comparison with placebo and/or another active agent is considered.[23] Confirmatory evidence could be obtained from non-invasive assessments. However, it is hoped that non-invasive ambulatory methods will improve such that the reverse may become true with the direct methods becoming confirmatory.

It is only with ambulatory techniques that the duration of action of a compound can be assessed accurately and from which sensible dosing regimens can be determined.[27,28] Design of studies to determine if a compound is an antihypertensive should be such that the effects of biological variability mentioned earlier can be minimised. Until now, this study design has always involved the use of the assessment of placebo, because it is well established that placebo has an 'effect' on reducing arterial pressure measured in the clinic.[26] However, evidence is growing that this may not be the case for direct[14] or non-invasive ambulatory monitoring techniques[5,9], although unfortunately Bellet et al.[3] did describe some effect of placebo with non-invasive ambulatory monitoring techniques. If there is no effect of placebo using ambulatory monitoring techniques, studies in antihypertensive patients can be simplified with this technique, with measurements before and after treatment being sufficient. This would cut the numbers of patients necessary to take part in studies, abolish the need for cross-over techniques and make statistical analysis easier. Perhaps if investigators used ambulatory techniques (especially non-invasive) to assess antihypertensive efficacy, a preliminary study to show lack of effect of placebo with techniques developed in their laboratories could provide useful information upon which to base subsequent studies.

Conclusion

The clinical measurement of arterial pressure plays an important part in the evaluation of new drugs, from the standpoint of safety (if the compound is not an antihypertensive agent) and of efficacy (if the compound is expected to affect arterial pressure). Methods to measure pressure have been developed over the past 100 years and have been more concerned with reducing factors known to produce variability in arterial pressure (which is inherent in human beings) than with new technology. The methods include the development not only of more sophisticated techniques, but also of the design of studies. The time has now arrived when the efficacy of an antihypertensive agent should include its effect in the clinic, the home and the workplace. Methods are now available to allow the collection of this information in order to make sensible assessments of new drugs to control hypertension.

References

[1] A.A.M.I. standard for electronic or automated sphygmomanometers. In *A.A.M.I. Standards*, V.A. Alington, Association for the Advancement of Medical Instrumentation, pp. 29–42, 1980.

[2] Arnold, J.M.O. and McDevitt, D.G. Indirect blood pressure measurement during intravenous isoprenaline infusions. *Brit. J. Clin. Pharmacol.*, 114–16, 1985.

[3] Bellet, M., Pagny, Y.L., Chatellier, G., Corvol, P., and Menard, J. Evaluation of slow release nicardipine in essential hypertension by casual and ambulatory blood pressure measurement. Effects of acute versus chronic administration. *J. Hypertension*, **5**, 597–604, 1987.

[4] Breit, S.N. and O'Rourke, M.F.O. Comparison of direct and indirect arterial pressure measurements in hospitalised patients. *Aust. N.Z. J. Med.*, **4**, 485–91, 1974.

[5] Conway, J., Johnston, J., Coats, A., Somer, V., and Sleight, P. The use of ambulatory monitoring to improve the accuracy and reduce the number of subjects in clinical trials of antihypertensive agents. *J. Hypertension*, **6**, 111–16, 1988.

[6] Corcoran, A.C., Dunstan, H.P., and Page, I.H. The evaluation of antihypertensive procedures, with particular reference to their effects on blood pressure. *ANN. Intern. Med.*, **43**, 1161–77, 1955.

[7] Cowan, R.M., Sokolow, M., and Perloff, D. Methodological consideration in determining the accuracy of an indirect blood pressure recorder. In *Isam 1979*, F.D. Stott, E.B. Raftery, and L. Goulding (eds), Academic Press Inc., London, 241–7, 1979.

[8] Dorlas, J.C., Nijboer, J.A., Butijn, W.T., Van der Hoeven, G.M.A., Selters, J.J., and Wesseling, H. Effects of peripheral vasoconstriction on the blood pressure in the finger measured continuously by a new non-invasive method (The Finapres). *Anaesthesiology*, **62**, 342–5, 1985.

[9] Dupont, A.G., Vandernienpen, P., and Six, R.O. Effect of Quanfacine on ambulatory blood pressure and its variability in elderly patients with essential hypertension. *Brit. J. Clin. Pharmacol.*, **23**, 397–401, 1987.

[10] Dupont, A.G., Vanderniepen, and Six, R.O. Placebo does not lower ambulatory blood pressure. *Brit. J. Clin. Pharmacol.*, **24**, 106–109, 1987.

[11] Fitzgerald, D.J., O'Malley, K., and O'Brien, E.T. Inaccuracy of London School of Hygiene sphygmomanometer. *Brit. Med. J.*, **284**, 18–20, 1982.

[12] Fitzgerald, D.J., O'Callaghan, W.G., McQuaid, R., O'Malley, K., and O'Brien, E.T. Accuracy and reliability of two indirect ambulatory blood pressure recorders: Remler M2000 and Cardiodyne Sphygmolog. *Brit. Heart. J.*, **48**, 572–9, 1982.

[13] Floras, J.S., Jones, J.V., Hassan, M.O., and Sleight, P. Ambulatory blood pressure during once-daily randomised double-blind administration of atenolol, metoprolol, pindolol and slow release propranolol. *Brit. Med. J.*, **285**, 1387–92, 1982.

[14] Gould, B.A., Mann, S., Davies, A.B., Altman, D.G., and Raftery, E.B. Does placebo lower blood pressure? *Lancet*, **ii**, 1377–81, 1981.

[15] Gould, B.A., Hornung, R.S., and Raftery, E.B. When should patients measure their blood pressure at home? A comparison of home and intra-arterial blood pressure. *J. Hypertension*, **1** (Supp. 2), 293–5, 1983.

[16] Harrington, K., Fitzgerald, P., O'Donnell, P., Hill, K.W., O'Brien, E.T., and O'Malley, K. Short and long-term treatment of essential hypertension with felodipine as monotherapy. *Drugs*, **34** (Supp. 3), 178–85, 1987.

[17] Harry, J.D. Clinical pharmacology of Epanolol. Pharmacodynamic aspects. *Drugs*, **38** (Supp. 2), 18–27, 1989.

[18] Harry, J.D. and Young, J. Preliminary experiences with the Remler M-2000; a semi-automatic indirect method for measuring blood pressure in ambulatory patients. In *Isam 1979*, F.D. Stott, E.B. Raftery, and L. Goulding (eds), Academic Press Inc., London, 215–22, 1979.

[19] Hill, L. and Barnard, H. A simple and accurate form of sphygmomanometer or arterial pressure gauge contrived for clinical use. *Brit. Med. J.*, **2**, 904, 1897.

[20] Julius, S., Ellis, C.N., Pascual, A.V., Matice, M., Hansson, L., Hun Yor, S.W., and Sandler, L.N. Home blood pressure determination: value in borderline ('labile') hypertension. *JAMA*, **229**, 663–6, 1974.

[21] Korotkoff, M.S. On the subject of methods of measuring blood pressure. *Bull. Imp. Military Med. Acad. St. Petersburg*, **11**, 365–7, 1905.

[22] Littler, W.A., Honover, A.J., Sleight, P., and Stott, F.D. Continuous recording of direct arterial pressure and electrocardiogram in unrestricted man. *Brit. Med. J.*, **3**, 76–8, 1972.

[23] Littler, W.A. and Komsuoghu, B. Which is the most accurate method of measuring blood pressure? *Am. Heart J.*, **117**, 723–8, 1989.

[24] Mancia, G., Bertinien, G., Grassi, G., Parati, G., Pomidossi, G., Ferrari, A., Gregorini, L., and Zanchetti, A. Effects of blood pressure measurement by the doctor on patients' blood pressure and heart rate. *Lancet*, **ii**, 695–7, 1983.

[25] Millar-Craig, M.W., Bishop, C.W., and Raftery, E.B. Circadian variation of blood pressure. *Lancet*, **i**, 795–7, 1978.

[26] Monstos, S.E., Supira, J.D., Scheib, E.T., and Shapiro, A.P. An analysis of the placebo effect in hospitalised hypertensive patients. *Clin. Pharmacol. Ther.*, **8**, 676–83 1967.

[27] O'Brien, E., Fitzgerald, D., and O'Malley, K. Blood pressure measurements: current practice and future trends. *Brit. Med. J.*, **290**, 729–34, 1985.

[28] O'Brien, E., Cox, J.P., and O'Malley, K. Ambulatory blood pressure measurement in the evaluation of blood pressure lowering drugs. *J. Hypertension*, **7**, 243–7, 1989.

[29] Parati, G., Casadei, R., Groppelli, A., DiRienzo, M., and Mancia, G. Comparison of finger and intra-arterial blood pressure monitoring at rest and during laboratory testing. *Hypertension*, **13**, 647–55, 1989.

[30] Petrie, J.C., O'Brien, E.T., Littler, W.A., and De Swiet, M. Recommendations on blood pressure measurement. *Brit. Med. J.*, **293**, 611–15, 1986.

[31] Pickering, G. and Stott, F.D. Ambulatory blood pressure – A review. In *Isam 1979*, F.D. Stott, E.B. Raftery, and L. Goulding (eds), Academic Press Inc., London, 135–45, 1979.

[32] Raftery, E.B. The methodology of blood pressure recording. *Brit. J. Clin. Pharmacol.*, **6**, 193–201, 1978.

[33] Raftery, E.B. and Ward, A.P. The indirect method of recording blood pressure. *Cardiovasc. Res.*, **2**, 210–18, 1968.

[34] Riva-Rocci, S. Un Nuovo Sfigmomanometro Gaz. *Med. Turino*, **47**, 981–96, 1986.

[35] Rose, G. The measurement of blood pressure. In *The Hypertensive Patient*, A.J. Marshall and D.V. Barritt (eds), Pitman Medical Limited, UK, 22–38, 1980.

[36] Waeber, G., Beck, G., Waeber, B., Bidiville, J., Nussberger, J., and

Brunner, H.R. Comparison of betaxolol with verapamil in hypertensive patients: discrepancy between office and ambulatory blood pressures. *J. Hypertension*, **6**, 239–45, 1988.

[37] White, W.B., Smith, V.E., McCabe, E.J., and Mieran, M.K. Effects of chronic nitrendipine on casual (office) and 24-hour ambulatory blood pressure. *Clin. Pharmacol. Ther.*, **38**, 60–4, 1985.

[38] Wright, B.M. and Dore, C.F. A random-zero sphygmomanometer. *Lancet*, **i**, 337–8, 1970.

5. Dose– and Concentration–Effect Relationships of Cardiovascular Drugs

B. Edgar and R. Bergstrand

Introduction

The clinical development of a drug includes the characterisation of the time-course of its plasma concentrations and those of its metabolites and their relationship to the intensity and duration of pharmacological effects. Differences in dynamic response within a patient population reflect individual variability in kinetics[25], variability due to differences between dosage forms[21], variability in compliance (see Chapter 10), and differences in sensitivity at receptor sites. Analysis should, therefore, be based on individual rather than mean results.[23]

This account illustrates the value of defining dose–concentration–effect relationships during the development of cardiovascular drugs and their pharmaceutical formulations.

Models

To define quantitative relationships between dose or plasma concentrations of a drug and response, various theoretical models are often used. These usually assume a reversible action of the drug at an effect site and that the measured concentration (usually in plasma) reflects the concentration at this site. The aim of chronic treatment may be the prevention of cardiovascular catastrophies, while the direct effect of the drug may be vasodilation resulting in reduction in blood pressure. It is often easier to describe a relationship between this direct effect (surrogate endpoint), rather than therapeutic effect, and dose or concentration.

One model that describes drug effects over the whole range of doses or concentrations is the 'E_{max} model', which predicts a hyperbolic relationship between the dose or concentration and the effect or change of effect (E).[13] It indicates no change in effect when no drug is present, and defines a maximum effect (E_{max}) (*Figure 5.1*) as well as the dose or concentration associated with 50% of the maximum effect (EC_{50}). If the baseline effect is stable and does not influence the drug effect, it can be subtracted from the measurements. In the case of antihypertensive drugs, blood pressure reduction is dependent on pre-treatment blood pressure. Baseline diastolic blood pressure (DBP) is

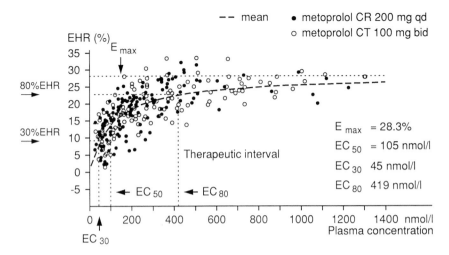

Figure 5.1. The concentration–effect relationship of metoprolol. EHR = exercise heart rate; E_{max} = maximal effect; EC_{50} = plasma drug concentration associated with 50% of the maximal effect. (From Abrahamsson *et al.*, 1990.[1])

usually between 90 and 115 mmHg in study populations and its distribution should be considered when interpreting results. In studies with felodipine, a linear relationship between pre-treatment DBP and the extent of drug effect was found when data from both healthy subjects and hypertensive patients were pooled.[3] Similar relationships have been found for other antihypertensive drugs.[26] Consideration of baseline values is therefore of great importance when seeking relationships between dose or concentration and effect.

The range of doses used or concentrations measured will determine which mathematical model to apply. Linear or log–linear correlations are usually easier to estimate than hyperbolic functions. The log–linear model is, therefore, commonly used to describe the relationship between dose or concentration and effect. In the range of 20–80% of the maximum effect, this relationship is a linear approximation of the E_{max} model. Simple linear or log–linear regressions can be used to describe the slope and intercepts and to make comparisons. However, by using non–linear regression methods applied to functions like the E_{max} model, maximum and minimum effect can also be evaluated. Furthermore, a therapeutic dose or concentration range may be estimated from the relationship (*Figure 5.1*).

Dose Ranging

In the first studies of a new chemical entity (NCE) in man, the need to establish the desired pharmacodynamic response has to be balanced against safety considerations. Based on the results from animal studies, escalating doses of a new substance are administered to healthy males. The desired pharmacological effect or a relevant surrogate endpoint is used to determine an anticipated minimum and maximum therapeutic dose. Assessments of the intensity and duration of pharmacodynamic effects as a function of dose are of great importance in the overall development of an NCE. The pharmacokinetic and dynamic data from these early studies will assist in the design of dosage regimens in subsequent patient studies. Initial dosing at the upper plateau of the dose–response curve may have serious consequences, since many adverse events are dose-related.[22] Many antihypertensive drugs have been introduced into the clinic in excessive doses based on results from studies in healthy subjects. This may reflect differential sensitivity to the drug in healthy and hypertensive subjects.

Since all drugs show intra- and inter-individual variations in effect, it is necessary to measure plasma drug concentrations to explain this variability and to understand the dose–concentration–effect relationship. If concentration–effect relationships are included in evaluations, a better understanding of the dose–response pattern can be achieved in studies with parallel group design.[4]

Dose–response studies are usually of parallel group design with fixed dosing in the different groups, and results are based on mean parameter estimates. As discussed by Sheiner et al.[23], this design does not disclose the influence of dosage increments in the individual patient. An excessive pharmacodynamic response may be the reason for a selective withdrawal of responders in higher dose groups, and the dose–response curve based on this kind of study design may therefore underestimate the effect of higher doses as well as the individual response to lower doses. The use of an hyperbolic model to describe the dose–response curve based either on individual or on mean population data, can contribute to a better understanding of the true dose–response pattern.[23]

Unwanted physiological effects may show dose–concentration–effect relationships other than the desired pharmacological effect and reduce the clinically acceptable dose range. For isradipine, the mean maximum decrease in DBP occurs at daily doses higher than 5 mg, above which adverse haemodynamic events increase more than additional antihypertensive effect.[24]

Examples

In one of the first studies in man of the calcium antagonist felodipine, intravenous doses ranging from 0.5 mg to 3.0 mg were given to ten healthy male subjects.[19] The effect on supine DBP and heart rate (HR) was dose-dependent, but of short duration. Because the mean half-life of felodipine was 3.6 h, the dosing interval in the first clinical studies was short and, because of low systemic availability, high oral doses were used.[11,17] The dose–response relationship in these early studies with felodipine was relatively flat, because dosing occurred at the plateau of the dose–response curve. Following additional dose–concentration–effect studies in healthy subjects and patients[12], doses were lowered dramatically in subsequent studies. The effect was better related to plasma drug concentration than to the dose. The therapeutic range of plasma felodipine concentration was found to be between 2–25 nmol/l, with the maximum possible effect, in patients with mild to moderate hypertension, being a decrease of DBP of about 25 mmHg.[10] In late phase III studies with felodipine, daily doses of 2.5–20 mg were used, compared with doses of up to 150 mg used in the early study by Leonetti *et al.*[17] Doses above 10 mg seemed to produce only small additional decreases in mean blood pressure.[5] Similar findings of a plateau in the dose–effect relationship for other antihypertensive drugs have been reported for beta-blockers.[23] The individual dose response may, however, be quite different from the mean result in a population.[4,23]

The relationship between plasma concentrations of metoprolol and its effect on exercise heart rate (EHR) was analysed in several studies using doses of 100–400 mg/day.[1] A lower effective concentration (30% of maximal reduction equal to a reduction in EHR of about 10 bpm) was estimated to be ~45 nM.[1] Concentrations above 300–400 nM, on the other hand, seemed to be associated with little additional beta-blockade (*Figure 5.1*).

Time Effect

The effect *versus* time curve plotted on the same graph as the concentration *versus* time curve may give information as to when to measure concentration and on the influence on effect of such factors as distribution, active metabolites and tolerance. Similarly, plots of effect as a function of consecutive concentrations (*Figure 5.2*) may give information about equilibration delays between plasma and receptor sites, formation of active metabolites or development of tolerance. These phenomena may also be disclosed if the relationship between concentration and effect changes with duration of treatment.

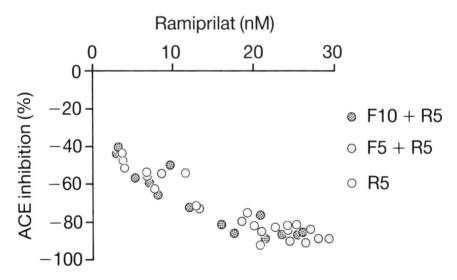

Figure 5.2. Inhibition of ACE activity *versus* plasma concentration of ramiprilat after ramipril 5 mg (R5) alone, and in combination with felodipine 5 mg (F5) and 10 mg (F10). (Mean data from 12 healthy subjects.) (From Bergstrand *et al.*, to be published.[2])

Examples

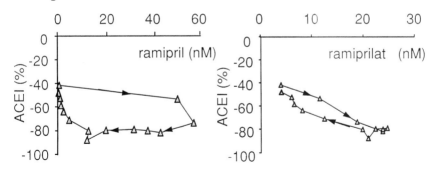

Figure 5.3. Inhibition of ACE activity (ACEI) *versus* plasma concentration of ramipril and ramiprilat. The arrows indicate the progress of concentrations with time. (From Bergstrand *et al.*, to be published.[2])

When the effect–time curve for metoprolol is plotted on the same time scale as the concentration–time curve, the peak concentration of metoprolol occurs at the same time as the maximum reduction in EHR.[1] Similar findings have been reported with regard to blood pressure and plasma concentrations of felodipine[22] and enalaprilat.[20] Thus, hysteresis is not seen, indicating a negligible delay in the equilibrium between drug concentration in plasma and at the site of action.

When a clockwise hysteresis is found, this may reflect a physiological adjustment to the effect of the drug, e.g. baroreceptor resetting in a vasodilator-dependent increase in heart rate.[9] The input rate of calcium antagonists has been shown to have a significant influence on the relationship between concentration and effect on diastolic blood pressure in healthy subjects.[6,16,27] This relationship may, however, be different in patients and healthy subjects as the baroreflex mediated increase in heart rate is less in hypertensive patients. A 'hysteresis' may indicate delayed distribution equilibrium or, as in the case of ramipril, the formation of the active substance (ramiprilat) from the prodrug (*Figure 5.3*). During prolonged treatment, formation of metabolites with agonistic or antagonistic activity, or the development of tolerance, may change the effect predicted from the first dose. Relationships between concentration and effect after single and multiple dosing must be shown to be similar in order to exclude the development of tolerance.[8,10]

Bioequivalence and Dynamic Equivalence

Immediate release formulations (IRF) and slow release formulations (SRF) of a drug are usually not bioequivalent because the latter exhibit lower C_{max} and t_{max} values and higher trough concentrations. However, pharmacodynamic effects may be similar if the high concentrations around C_{max} after an IRF have reached the plateau of the concentration–effect curve. Furthermore, the total effect over 24 hours after an SRF may be similar or higher because of less fluctuation in the concentration–time course.

Table 5.1. A comparison of mean pharmacokinetic and pharmacodynamic parameters after different doses and formulations of metoprolol (from Lücher et al.[18])

Dose/day (mg)		Slow release formulation (SRF)			Immediate release formulation (IRF)		
	Admin.	AUC* (nM h)	AUEC† (% h)	Admin.		AUC* (nM h)	AUEC† (% h)
100	100 od	2433‡	206	100 od		2934‡	173
200	200 od	5843‡	438	100 bid		7876‡	428
300	300 od	12368‡	547	100 tid		16860‡	582
400	400 od	12920‡	527	100 qid		15481‡	541

* AUC = Area under the plasma drug concentration–time curve.
† AUEC = Area under the effect–time curve (reduction in exercise tachycardia).
‡ Significant difference between IRF and SRF.

A pharmacokinetic comparison of a new SRF of metoprolol with a conventional IRF (*Table 5.1*) showed a decreased availability (80%) of the slow release formulation. However, the total effect over 24 hours on exercise heart rate was no different.[18] Thus, the formulations were pharmacodynamically equivalent when the SRF was administered once daily and the IRF was given in divided doses.

Interactions

The co-administration of two drugs with different mechanisms of action may produce an additive or synergistic effect due to pharmacodynamic or kinetic interactions. The concentration–effect relationship may be more complex than that for each individual compound, with additive or synergistic effects at lower concentrations[13], while higher concentrations may impair the effectiveness of the combination. Multifactorial studies with several dose combinations have been proposed as the experimental design of choice to evaluate the effect of drug combinations.[14]

Concentration–effect relationships may be influenced by metabolites formed during the first pass. Intravenous administration may therefore give rise to a different relationship between concentration and effect than does an oral administration. Metabolites formed and accumulated during multiple administration may produce different drug–effect relationships from those seen after single doses.

Drug–Drug Interactions

The main effect of ACE inhibitors is a reduction in the concentration of angiotensin II. A relationship between this reduction and plasma concentrations of enaprilat and ramiprilat has been shown.[2,20] Calcium antagonists, on the other hand, activate the renin–angiotensin system and possibly increase angiotensin II levels. Although a combination of ACE inhibitor and calcium antagonist may produce a favourable blood pressure reduction, the effect on angiotensin levels may be complex. The addition of felodipine (5 or 10 mg) to the ACE inhibitor ramipril, however, did not change the relationship between the plasma concentration of ramiprilat and reduction of angiotensin II activity (*Figure 5.2*).[2]

The addition of a calcium antagonist to a beta-blocker may cause an additive antihypertensive effect, due to changes in plasma concentrations of the beta-blocker and because of the different mechanisms of action and agonistic effects on sympathetic activity. Such a beneficial interaction has been shown for felodipine and metoprolol.[7] However, neither dose– nor concentration–effect relationships of the combination have been evaluated.

Drug Metabolite

If the relationship between plasma drug concentration and effect is similar after acute intravenous and oral administration, it is likely that no metabolite with the same pharmacodynamic effect is formed during the first pass. On the other hand, if such metabolites are formed, the relationship will be route-dependent, as shown with quinidine.[13] As quinidine forms several metabolites, concentration–effect relationships are complex. It seems that concentrations of the 3-OH metabolite are better related to changes in conduction than are those of quinidine itself.[15]

Summary

A well-defined prospective use of dose–concentration–effect relationships of an NCE or a new formulation will reduce the total number of subjects and patients needed to define the therapeutic dosage regimen. Furthermore, these data help to evaluate intra- as well as inter-individual variability and thereby rationalise the range of unit dose sizes required.

In addition, an analysis of effect as a function of time during and after drug administration, producing a wide range of plasma concentrations, will guide the development of better dosage forms.

Dose–concentration–effect data obtained after co-administration of drugs will improve our understanding of drug–drug interactions and the development of rational combination products.

References

[1] Abrahamsson, B., Lücher, P., Olofsson, B., Regual, C.G., Sandberg, A., Wieselgren, L., and Bergstrand, R. The relationship between metoprolol pharma concentration and beta-blockade in healthy subjects: a study on conventional metopronol and metapronol CR/ZOK formulations. *J. Clin. Pharmacol.*, **30**, 546–54, 1990.

[2] Bergstrand, R., Edgar, B., and Skiöldebrand, E. A comparative study of ramipril in combination with different doses of felodipine (to be published).

[3] Blychert, E., Edgar, B., Elmfeldt, D., and Hedner, T. Blood pressure response of felodipine and its relation to concentration in a large population (to be published).

[4] Brun, J. and Edgar, B. Dos respons i kontrollerad versus öppen studie med felodipine (to be published).

[5] Brun, J., Fröberg, L., Kronmann, P., Olsson, L-B., Skoog, P., Tygesen, G., Bengtsson, C., Schevsten, B., and Tieblin, G. Optimal felodipine dose when combined with metaprolol in arterial hypertension: a Swedish multicentre study within primary health care. *J. Cardiovasc. Pharmacol.*, **15** (Suppl. 4), 560–4, 1990.

[6] Cohen, A.F., van Hall, M., van Harten, J., and Breimer, D.D. Effects of different infusion rates of felodipine on haemodynamic and baroreflex sensitivity. *Clin. Pharmacol. Ther.*, **47**, 1422, 1990.

[7] Dahlöf, B. and Hosie, J. Antihypertensive efficacy and tolerability of a fixed combination of metoprolol and felodipine in comparison with the individual substances in monotherapy. *J. Cardiovasc. Pharmacol.*, **16**, 910–6, 1990.

[8] Donnelly, R., Elliot, H.L., Meredith, P.A., and Reid, J.L. Acute and chronic nifedipin in essential hypertension: concentration–effect relationship. *Clin. Sci.*, **73**, 54, 1987.

[9] Dunselman, P.H.J.M. *Felodipine Congestive Heart Failure*, Thesis, Gröningen, 1989.

[10] Edgar, B. Clinical pharmacokinetics of felodipine, Thesis, University of Göthenborg, 1988.

[11] Elmfeldt, D. and Hedner, T. Felodipine, a new vasodilator, in addition to beta-blockade in hypertension. *Eur. J. Clin. Pharmacol.*, **25**, 571–5, 1983.

[12] Elmfeldt, D. and Edgar, B. The relation between plasma concentration of felodipine and effect on diastolic blood pressure. Hässle Report, Mölndal, Sweden, 1987.

[13] Holford, N.H. and Sheiner, L.B. Understanding the dose–effect relationship: clinical application of pharmacokinetic pharmacodynamic models. *Clin. Pharmacokinetics*, **6**, 429–53, 1981.

[14] Johnsson, G. and Lörstad, M. The scientific justification for fixed combination therapy. *Proc. Eur. Soc. Regulatory Affairs*, 1988.

[15] Kavanagh, K.M., Wyse, G.D., Mitchell, L.B., Gilhooly, T., Gillis, A., and Duff, H. Contribution of quinide metabolites to electrophysiologic response in human subjects. *Clin. Pharmacol. Ther.*, **46**, 352–8, 1989.

[16] Kleinbloesem, C.H., van Brummeln, P., Danhof, M., Faber, H., Urquhart, J., and Breimer, D.D. Rate of increase in the plasma concentration of nifedipine as a major determinant of its haemodynamic effect in humans. *Clin. Pharmacol.*, **41**, 26–30, 1987.

[17] Leonetti, G., Gradnick, R., Terzoli, L., Fruscio, M., and Rupoli, L. Felodipine, a new vasodilating drug: blood pressure, cardiac, renal and humoral effects in hypertensive patients. *J. Cardiovasc. Pharmacol.*, **6**, 392–8, 1984.

[18] Lücker, P., Moore, G., Wieselgren, I., Olofsson, B., and Bergstrand, R. Pharmacokinetic and pharmacodynamic comparison of metoprol Cr/zon once daily with conventional tablets over dosing and in divided doses. *J. Clin. Pharmacol.*, **30**, 517–77, 1990.

[19] Lundborg, P. and Edgar, B. A study of the safety and tolerance after an escalating single dose of felodipine (H154/82). *Hässle Report V–104*, Mölndal, Sweden, 1983.

[20] Meredith, P.A., Elliot, H.L., Donnelly, R., and Reid, J.L. Prediction and optimisation of enalapril (ENC) therapy in hypertension. *Clin. Pharmacol. Ther.*, **97**, 151, 1990.

[21] Peck, C. The randomised concentration-controlled clinical trial (CCT): an information-rich alternative to the randomised placebo-controlled clinical trial (PCT). *Clin. Pharmacol. Ther.*, **47**, 148, 1990.

[22] Reid, J. Dose–plasma concentration–effect relationship for felodipine in essential hypertension: a review. *Cardiovasc. Pharmacol.*, **15** (Suppl. 4), 550–6, 1990.

[23] Sheiner, L.W., Beal, S.L., and Sambol, N.C. Study design for dose ranging. *Clin. Pharmacol. Ther.*, **46**, 63–77, 1989.

[24] Simonsen, K. and Sundqvist, K.D. Dose–response relationship and incidence of adverse drug reactions with isradipine in patients with essential hypertension. *Am. J. Med.*, **1986** (Suppl. 4A), 91–3, 1989.

[25] Sjöqvist, F. Inter-individual difference in drug responses: an overview. In *Variability in Drug Therapy,* Rowland *et al.* (eds), Raven Press, New York, 1–9, 1985.

[26] Summer, D.J., Meredith, P.A., Howie, C.A., Elliot, H.L., and Reid, J.C. Initial blood pressure as a predictor of the response to antihypertensive therapy. *Br. J. Clin. Pharmacol.*, **26**, 715–20, 1988.

[27] van Harten, J., Burggraaf, J., Ligthart, G.J., van Brummelen, P., and Briemer, D.D. Single and multiple dose kinetics and effects in the young, the middle-aged, and the elderly. *Clin. Pharmacol. Ther.*, **45**, 600–7, 1989.

6. Rating Scales in Psychiatry: Uses in the Assessment of Drug Effects

L.F. Gram

Introduction

Since the breakthrough in psychopharmacology 30–35 years ago with the introduction of neuroleptics, antidepressants, lithium and benzodiazepines, further developments have been rather slow with no genuine innovations. The drugs used today are generally based on the prototypes developed in the 1950s and 1960s. However, there are several good reasons for seeking to develop better psychotropic drugs. For example, the incomplete effect of neuroleptics, particularly on core schizophrenia symptoms, such as autism, and their disturbing side effects, in particular Parkinsonism and tardive dyskinesia, leaves considerable room for improvement. Likewise, the tricyclic antidepressants are not ideal, because of their slow onset of action, the relatively high frequencies of treatment resistance and drop-outs due to intolerable side effects, and their overdose toxicity. The 'second-generation' antidepressants developed during the past 10–20 years have only gained limited acceptance, largely because of questionable efficacy compared to the tricyclics.[17,18,44,57] The use of lithium is also limited by side effects and toxicity, and a dependence and abuse liability is a potential problem with most benzodiazepines.

The considerable investment made by the pharmaceutical industry during the past 10–20 years in developing new and better psychotropic drugs is clearly justified, but innovations have been difficult for several reasons. Despite the considerable resources invested in biological psychiatry research over the past 25 years, progress has been rather disappointing[56]:

- No specific biological index of mental disease has been found.
- The biological etiologies of mental diseases are not known with any certainty.
- Reliable diagnostic or predictive biological tests have not been developed.
- The biological basis of the mode of action of psychotropic drugs is largely unknown.

Psychotropic Drug Development

The development of new psychotropic drugs thus poses problems both at the pre-clinical hypothesis-generating level and on the clinical side where all

assessments of new drugs have to rely on non-biological clinical measurements. The effect measurement is, however, only one of several problems in
the clinical testing of new psychotropic drugs. The basic principles of
randomisation and blinding have gained general acceptance in clinical
psychopharmacology in parallel with developments in other fields of clinical
pharmacology. Although statistical considerations underlying the calculation
of sample size are generally accepted, many studies still include far too few
patients. The risk of Type II statistical error is compounded by uncertainty
about the dose–effect relationship for both control and test drugs, compliance
problems, high rates of spontaneous response, poor patient selection, and
other deficiencies in the conduct of studies.[25] The development of rating
scales and diagnostic inventories has now reached a high scientific level[51],
and, provided that validated tests are used carefully and with regular control
measures, this aspect of assessment is no longer a major problem.[25]

Methods of Evaluation in Clinical Psychopharmacology

The development of rating scales and diagnostic inventories started early in
psychiatry[11,26,30,31,36,41,53], and the basic principles have subsequently been
adopted in other areas of clinical pharmacology, where it has been realised
that the availability of biological effect measurements does not necessarily
guarantee valid and reliable results.

The methods of evaluation developed in psychiatry[51] attempt to measure
several factors in relation to disease (diagnosis, symptom profile, severity),
personality, life events, quality of life, social adaptation, interpersonal
interactions and non-therapeutic drug effects (side effects, adverse reactions,
dependence) (*Table 6.1*).

Table 6.1.

Type of evaluation	Selected references
Diagnostic inventories	2, 15, 27, 37
Severity rating:	
Comprehensive scales	4, 16, 19, 23, 33, 46
Schizophrenia/psychoses	3, 40, 41
Depression	5, 11, 29, 39, 58
Mania	10, 13, 54
Aggression	42, 55
Anxiety	30, 48, 49
Obsessive–compulsive disorder	45, 50
Dementia, cognitive dysfunction	24
Personality	14, 22, 31, 34
Child behaviour	1
Mental retardation	12
Social adaptation	20, 21, 52
Quality of life	38
Life events	32, 43
Drug side effects/adverse reactions	35, 47

The content of the scales may serve *diagnostic* or *quantitative* purposes, and the scales may be *comprehensive* or *specific* (syndrome related).

The *construction* may be based on *global assessment* or on *items* relating to specific symptoms.

The *assessment* is based on either *observer rating* (psychiatrist, nurse, psychologist) or patient *self-rating*.

As shown in *Table 6.1*, the high level of activity in this field throughout the past 20–30 years has resulted in a variety of rating-assessments for most diseases or malfunctions in psychiatry and related disciplines. For some conditions, such as depression, the number of available scales is very large and it is important to select scales with due consideration of quality, relevance and applicability.[51] Generally, the use of global scales can be considered only as a supplement, whereas the documentation of drug effects ought to be based on well-established rating scales.

The proper evaluation of a rating scale should take several dimensions into account[51], the most important being *validity, reliability, applicability, sensitivity* (to change) and *informative value*.

The Validity of Rating Scales

The *validity* of a scale, i.e., the extent to which it measures what it is meant to measure, is a fundamental attribute, but one which is the most difficult to assess.

Face validity reflects the extent to which the symptom items included in the scale can be considered as clinically meaningful measures of the disease or syndrome in question.

Construct validity usually refers to the theoretical basis of the construction of a scale.

External or concurrent validity refers to the degree to which a quantitative measurement obtained on a rating scale correlates with some other measurement of the same disease. In the absence of biological measurements, global clinical assessment of severity has often been used.[6,7] A typical rating scale, such as the Hamilton Depression Rating Scale (HDS)[30] (*Table 6.2*), includes a series of items by which individual symptoms are rated on an ordinal scale. Each score on each item should be carefully defined in a manual and, ideally, the items should be constructed such that the scale becomes an interval scale.

Table 6.2. Hamiltonian depression rating scale.[28]

Depressed mood	(0–4)	Anxiety psychic	(0–4)
Guilt feeling	(0–4)	Anxiety somatic	(0–4)
Suicidal	(0–4)	Gastrointestinal	(0–2)
Insomnia { initial	(0–2)	Somatic general	(0–2)
middle	(0–2)	Sexual interest	(0–2)
late	(0–2)	Hypochondria	(0–4)
Work and interest	(0–4)	Insight	(0–2)
Retardation	(0–4)	Weight loss	(0–2)
Agitation	(0–4)		
		TOTAL	(0–52)

Although the latter is difficult to substantiate, it does form an implicit basis for using the *total score* as a measure of total severity. Furthermore, the basis for this procedure is that the collection of items represents one entity and that the relative weighting of the different items is relevant. Validation against a global clinical assessment permits the analysis of several properties of the single item.[7] The correlation should exhibit *ascending monotonicity* and the absence of this for several items appears to explain why the total HDS score cannot differentiate between moderate and severe depression as rated on a global assessment.[7] Validation against global assessment carries a risk of circular conclusions. In fact, reversing the analysis, by looking at the items co-varying with high global score, may be a procedure for evaluating the global rater's conception of the disease syndrome in question (judgement analysis[8,9]).

Predictive validity refers to the ability of the rating scale to predict the course of the disease or the effect of treatment. In principle, only diagnostic scales are appropriate for such predictions. Even extensive item analysis has not been very successful in predicting the outcome of treatment in schizophrenia or depression. On the other hand, the changes in severity rating scores during treatment, and the differences between placebo and active treatment in this respect, can afford good proof of the validity of the scales employed.

Consistency of a scale[6,26] refers to how the items of a scale mutually agree (homogeneity) and how the scoring is independent of disease-independent variables, such as sex, social status, etc. (transferability). Homogeneity and transferability of a given scale can be tested by the Rash models.[6] Implicit in the consistency concept is reliability.[6]

Reliability of Rating Scales

Reliability refers to the *reproducible* and *unbiased* use of the rating scales. Reliability is a prerequisite for the validity of the rating measurement.

Reproducibility is usually considered in relation to the observation of the same patients by several raters, or by one rater several times. Statistical evaluation usually involves the calculation of intraclass correlations.[5]

Bias influencing the scoring on individual items may have several sources:

- *Logical error*: the rater's concept of the disease or syndrome is deviant and inconsistent with the scale construction.
- *Halo-effect*: the rater's global impression of the patient influences the scoring.
- *Central tendency*: untrained raters tend to avoid scoring at the extremes of the scale.
- *Congruence/contrast*: the rater's personal feelings, opinions, sympathies and antipathies influence the scoring on some items.

In clinical studies, high reliability with respect to both reproducibility and bias is maintained by general and specific training of the raters and by regular joint rating sessions.

Rating Scales in Psychotropic Drug Evaluation

The choice of rating scale is important and should take account of the validity and reliability considerations discussed above. Variations in the quality of different scales may be marginal in evaluating some conditions, such as depression, whereas in others, where difficulties in assessment are considerable, such as dementia, the choice of rating scale may be critical. As an example of the former case, data from a study comparing the selective 5-hydroxytryptamine (5HT)-reuptake inhibitor paroxetine with imipramine and placebo in the treatment of depression are shown in *Table 6.3*.[44] The intermediate efficacy of paroxetine is reflected homogeneously by all three rating scales and by all three of the global scales employed.

The *applicability* of rating scales relates in particular to their length and the definitions of the items. The customary use of several similar rating scales (*Table 6.3*) may be impractical if the same items on different scales cannot be merged because the scoring systems differ.[30,39] Since the total time available for completing a rating scale is limited, the inclusion of several similar scales and the use of extensive documentation should be balanced against the need for carefully conducted and valid ratings.

Global scales[16,28] are easy to apply, but difficulty in validation and their low information content limit their relevance, and such a scale should not be the only rating scale used. It has been claimed that global scales are sometimes more sensitive than other rating scales, but this may as much reflect shortcomings of the other scales used. Self-rating scales[11,58] may be useful in assessing some conditions, such as anxiety[48], whereas their applicability in severely depressed, psychotic or demented patients is limited.

The *sensitivity to change* may vary for different scales. Whereas the differences between the established depression scales are marginal, the scales for conditions such as schizophrenia or dementia may vary considerably in this respect.[24,40,41] Drug treatment in these latter conditions is characterised by having effect on only a fraction of the total psychopathology. Because of noise from residual symptoms, a beneficial drug effect may be difficult to

Table 6.3.

	TCA* (imipramine)	SSRI† (paroxetine)	Placebo
Rating scales:			
Hamilton DS	16	10	4
MADRS	17	12	5
Raskin DS	4.4	2.8	1.6
Global scales:			
CGI	1.8	1.0	0.5
MD–Global	1.7	1.3	0.3
Pat.–Global	1.7	1.1	0.2

* TCA: Tricyclic antidepressant.
† SSRI: Selective 5HT-reuptake inhibitor.

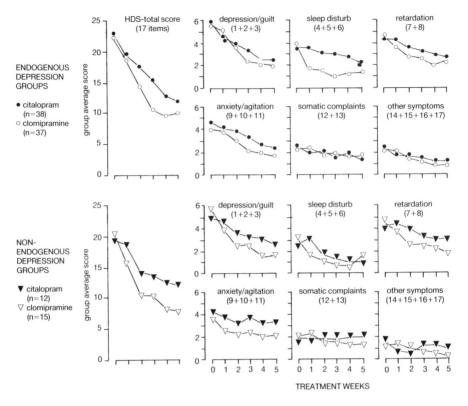

Figure 6.1. Group average scores on a total 17-item Hamilton Depression Rating Scale (HDS)[30] and clusters of HDS in patients treated with citalopram and clomipramine.[17]

detect unless a more selective subscale is used. Reducing the number of 'drug sensitive' items may, however, lower the sensitivity of the total score.

The use of *rating scale measurements* of drug effects raises several questions:

- Should *total score, subscale (cluster) score* or *single item scores* be used?
- Should *changes in score* or *final score* be used?
- Should the score be given in *absolute* values or *relative* values (relative to initial score)?
- Should data be analysed and presented as group-average scores or distributed according to classification of the patients into response categories?

It has been customary in psychotropic drug trials to concentrate on total scores in accordance with attempts to develop scales with a high degree of homogeneity. The use of total scores, on a homogeneous scale, will also for statistical reasons usually represent a more sensitive measure of changes. However, in the evaluation of new drugs, qualitative as well as quantitative differences may be of interest. Therefore, as shown in *Figure 6.1*, it is often relevant to perform separate analyses of clusters of items representing different parts of the complete syndrome. In this comparison between the selective 5HT-reuptake inhibitors citalopram and clomipramine[17], a better antidepressive effect was found with the latter, this difference appearing to involve all major components of the depressive syndrome. The only indication of a qualitative difference was the more pronounced sleep-restoring effect of clomipramine in the first week. The general homogeneity of the HDS is also demonstrated by the uniform results in the two diagnostic sub-groups (endogenous, non-endogenous)[15,27].

The question of whether to use the change in score (amelioration score) or the final score, and the use of absolute or relative measures, has been the subject of considerable debate. If the initial score is A and the final score is B, the possible measurements of drug effect are: $(A - B)$, B, $(A - B)/A$, or B/A. Conceptually, the amelioration score $(A - B)$ seems to reflect the drug effect most closely, but the importance of the initial score may make this measure less clinically relevant than the final score (B). Likewise, the relative measurements $[(A - B)/A]$ or B/A may be invalidated to some degree by the strong influence of the initial score. However, the different measures usually correlate quite well and it becomes a matter of taste as to which is chosen.[18,44]

Separate analysis of single items is usually required when the different items record independent unrelated symptoms. Comprehensive scales[4,20,23,37] and side effect scales[35] ought to be analysed in this way, and the principle may also be employed with more homogeneous scales, at least when more pronounced differences between treatments are expected (e.g. in placebo-controlled studies). *Table 6.4* shows results obtained with the UKU-side effect scale[35] in a recent study comparing paroxetine and clomipramine.[18] A comprehensive side effect scale was used which included several depression-

Table 6.4.

Symptoms (item nos. on the UKU scale[35]		Paroxetine (P)*	Clomipramine (C)*	Drug difference in final rating score (weeks)†
Impaired concentration	(1.1)	↓	↓	C < P (4, 6)
Disturbed memory	(1.4)	↓	↓	C < P (4)
Depression	(1.5)	↓	↓	C < P (4)
Tension/restlessness	(1.6)	↓	↓	C < P (2, 4, 6)
Sleep length reduced	(1.8)	↓	↓	C < P (2)
Headache	(4.17)	–	↓	C < P (2, 4, 6)
Asthenia	(1.2)	↓	↓	–
Emotional difference	(1.10)	↓	↓	–
Weight loss	(4.6)	↓	↓	–
Tremor	(2.5)	–	↑	C > P (4, 6)
Dry mouth	(3.3)	–	↑	C > P (2, 4, 6)
Orthostatic dizziness	(3.9)	–	↑	–
Increased sweating	(3.11)	–	↑	–

* ↓ : Reduction in score, i.e. improvement; ↑ : Increase in score, i.e. worsening; –: Unchanged (analysis based on contingency table and Fisher's exact test (significance level: 0.05), comparing pretreatment and treatment ratings).
† Fisher's exact test (significance level: 0.05); weeks of active treatment given in parenthesis.

Table 6.5.

	Study 1		Study 2	
	Citalopram	Clomipramine	Paroxetine	Clomipramine
Group average HDS	13.2	9.2	14.6	10.0
Responders (HDS<7) (%)	22	49	15	28
Partial responders (HDS 8–15) (%)	39	35	40	58
Non-responders (HDS≥16) (%)	39	16	45	14

related items. It can be seen that several of these symptoms declined in intensity, probably reflecting the antidepressant effect of the drugs. The better antidepressive effect of clomipramine was reflected by these single item analyses. True side effects, i.e. reflected in an increase in rating score, were only seen with clomipramine on items representing typical side effects of tricyclic antidepressants.

Finally, the preference for group average scores as opposed to response categories is also quite arbitrary. When the treatment differences are clear, the two measurements yield much the same conclusion (*Table 6.5*). The category response assessment may be considered to be more meaningful clinically, but the use of total scores for defining response categories may also weaken the statistical power of assessment.[17,18] In other conditions, such as schizophrenia, where only partial restoration can be expected, it may be meaningless to define response categories as is done in research on antidepressants.

The *informative value* of a rating score refers to its clinical meaning, as discussed above, and to its role as a means for *scientific communication*. When an antidepressant is reported to cause a decline in the group average total score on the HDS 17-item scale to about 10 after four weeks' treatment, most researchers in the field would know that this was a reasonably good overall response. However, when the score on the *XX* scale is reported to be reduced to less than *YY* in *ZZ*% of the patients, the reader might have considerable difficulty in translating this information into something meaningful. There is a need for an internationally accepted 'yardstick', and therefore it is often recommended that a well-established scale is included in the rating battery. Alternatively, if a new scale is used, some kind of conversion factor should be given, although this may require separate correlation studies.

Conclusion

In the absence of reliable, biological measurements of morbidity or drug effects, drug research in psychiatry has always depended on the use of so-called rating scales. These are based on semi-quantitative assessment of symptoms or signs (items) related to depression, acute psychoses, anxiety, etc. A key factor is the use of a total score for clusters or for all items on a scale. The validity of this may be tested against independent (global) measurements, effect of treatments, etc. The reliability of the scales depends on their construction, item definition, and rater experience and training. Over 30 years' experience with such scales has shown that they are reasonably accurate and sensitive for recording drug effects, provided the quality of the rating procedures is maintained. Currently, effect measurements are *not* the greatest problem in the assessment of putative, psychotropic drugs. Of more importance is the design and conduct of trials. In particular, the combined effects of high rates of spontaneous response and high rates of underdosing, owing to poor compliance or the use of inappropriate doses, explain problems related to Type II statistical errors.

References

[1] Achenbach, T. *Manuals of the Child Behaviour Checklist and Revised Child Behaviour*. University Associates in Psychiatry, Burlington, Vermont, 1988.

[2] American Psychiatric Association. *Diagnostical and Statistical Manual of Mental Disorders,* 3. Revision-revised (DSM–III–R). American Psychiatric Association Press, Washington DC, 1987.

[3] Andreassen, N.C. and Olsen, S. Negative versus positive schizophrenia. Definition and validation. *Arch. Gen. Psych.*, **39**, 789–94, 1982.

[4] Åsberg, M., Perris, C., Schalling, D., and Sedvall, G. The CPRS-development and applications of a psychiatric rating scale. *Acta Psychiatrica Scand.*, **58** (Suppl. 271), 1978.

[5] Bartko, J.J. and Carpenter, W.T. On the methods and theory of reliability. *J. Nervous Mental Disorders*, **163**, 307–17, 1976.

[6] Bech, P. Rating scales for affective disorders. Their validity and consistency. *Acta Psychiatrica Scand.*, **64** (Suppl. 295), 1981.

[7] Bech, P., Gram, L.F., Dein, E., Jacobsen, O., Vitger, J., and Bolwig, T.G. Quantitative rating of depressive states. *Acta Psychiatrica Scand.*, **51**, 161–70, 1975.

[8] Bech, P., Haaber, A., Joyce, C.B.R., and Danish University Antidepressant Group (DUAG). Experiments on clinical observations and judgement in the assessment of depression. *Psychol. Med.*, **16**, 873–83, 1986.

[9] Bech, P. and Rafaelsen, O.J. The melancholia scale: development, consistency, validity and utility. In *Assessment of Depression*, N. Sartorius and T.A. Ban (eds), Springer, Berlin, pp 259–69, 1986.

[10] Bech, P., Rafaelsen, O.J., Kramp, P., and Bolwig, T.G. The mania rating scale. Scale construction and inter-observer agreement. *Neuropharm.*, **17**, 430–1, 1978.

[11] Beck, A.T., Ward, C.H., Mendelson, M., Mock, J., and Erbaugh, J. An inventory for measuring depression. *Arch. Gen. Psych.*, **4**, 561–71, 1961.

[12] Bernsen, A.H. The children's handicaps, behaviour and skills (HBS) schedule. *Acta Psychiatrica Scand.*, **62** (Suppl. 285), 133–9, 1980.

[13] Biegel, A., Murphy, D.L., and Bunney, W.E. The manic-state rating scale. *Arch. Gen. Psych.*, **25**, 256–62, 1971.

[14] Bond, M., Gardner, S.T., Christian, J., and Sigal, J.J. Empirical study of self-rated defence styles. *Arch. Gen. Psych.*, **40**, 333–8, 1983.

[15] Carney, M.W.P., Roth, M., and Garside, R.F. The diagnosis of depressive syndromes and the prediction of ECT response. *Br. J. Psych.*, **111**, 659–74, 1965.

[16] CGI – Clinical Global Impressions. In *ECDEU Assessment Manual for Psychopharmacology*, W.D. Guy (ed). Revised 1976. US Department of Health, Education and Welfare, Public Health Service; Alcohol, Drug Abuse, and Mental Health Administration. DHEW Publication No. 76–338, 1976.

[17] Danish University Antidepressant Group (DUAG). Citalopram: clinical effect profile in comparison with clomipramine. *Psychopharm.*, **90**, 131–8, 1986.

[18] Danish University Antidepressant Group (DUAG). Paroxetine – a selective serotonin reuptake inhibitor showing better tolerance, but weaker antidepressant effect than clomipramine in a controlled multicentre study. *J. Affective Disorders*, **18**, 289–99, 1990.

[19] Derogatis, L.R. The psychosocial adjustment to illness scale. *Psychosomatic Res.*, **26**, 11–22, 1982.

[20] Derogatis, L.R. and Cleary, P. Confirmation of the dimensional structure of the SCL-90: a study in construct validation. *J. Clin. Psychol.*, **33**, 981–9, 1977.

[21] Endicott, J., Spitzer, R.L., Fleiss, J.L., and Cohen, J. The Global Assessment Scale. *Arch. Gen. Psych.*, **33**, 766–71, 1976.

[22] Eysenck, H.J. and Eysenck, S.B.G. *Manual of the Eysenck Personality Questionnaire*. Hodder and Stoughton, London, 1985.

[23] Goldberg, D. and Williams, P.A. *User's Guide to the General Health Questionnaire*, NFER-Nelson, Windsor, 1988.

[24] Gottfries, C.G., Bråne, G., and Steen, G. A new rating scale for dementia syndromes. *Gerontology* (Suppl. 2), 20–31, 1982.

[25] Gram, L.F. Inadequate dosing and pharmacodynamic variability as confounding factors in assessment of efficacy of antidepressants. *Clin. Neuropharm.*, **13** (Suppl. 1), 35–43, 1990.

[26] Guildford, J.P. *Psychometric Methods*, 2nd edition. McGraw-Hill Publishing Company, London, 1954.

[27] Gurney, C. *Diagnostic scales for affective disorders*. Proc. 5th World Conference of Psychiatry, Mexico City, p 130, 1971.

[28] Guy, W. *Clinical Global Impressions*. Early Clinical Drug Evaluation Unit (ECDEU) – National Institute of Health, 218–22, 1976.

[29] Hamilton, M. The assessment of anxiety states by rating. *Br. J. Med. Psychol.*, **32**, 50–5, 1959.

[30] Hamilton, M. Development of a rating scale for primary depressive illness. *Br. J. Sociol. Clin. Psychol.*, **6**, 278–96, 1967.

[31] Hathaway, S.R. and McKinley, J.C. *Minnesota Multiphasic Personality Inventory*. The Psychological Corporation, New York, 1951.

[32] Holmes, T.H. and Rahe, R.H. The Social Readjustment Rating Scale. *J. Psychosomatic Res.*, **11**, 213–18, 1967.

[33] Honigfeld, G. NOSIE-30: history and current status of its use in pharmacopsychiatric research. In *Psychological Measurements in Psychopharmacology. Modern Problems in Pharmacopsychiatry*, Vol. 7, P. Pichot (ed), Karger, Basel, pp 238–63, 1974.

[34] Hyler, S.E., Rieder, R.O., Williams, J.B.W., Spitzer, R.L., Hendler, J., and Lyons, M. The personality diagnostic questionnaire: development and preliminary results. *J. Personal Disorders*, **2**, 229–37, 1988.

[35] Lingjaerde, O., Ahlfors, U.G., Bech, P., Dencker, S-J., and Elgen, K. The UKU-side effect rating scale. *Acta Psychiatrica Scand.*, **76** (Suppl. 334), 1–100, 1987.

[36] Lorr, M. Rating scales and check lists for the evaluation of psychopathology. *Psychological Bull.*, **51**, 119–27, 1954.

[37] Lorr, M., Klett, C.J., McNair, C.M., and Lasky, J.J. *Inpatient Multidimensional Psychiatric Scale.* Consulting Psychologist Press, Palo Alto, 1963.

[38] Malm, U., May, P.R.A., and Dencker, S.J. Evaluation of the quality of life of the schizophrenic outpatient: a checklist. *Schizophrenia Bull.*, **7**, 1477–87, 1981.

[39] Montgomery, S.A. and Åsberg, M. A new depression scale designed to be sensitive to change. *Br. J. Psych.*, **134**, 382–9, 1979.

[40] Montgomery, S.A., Taylor, P. and Montgomery, D. Development of a schizophrenia scale sensitive to change. *Neuropharm.*, **17**, 1061–3, 1978.

[41] Overall, J.E. The brief psychiatric rating scale in psychopharmacology research. *Mod. Prob. Pharmacopsychiatry*, **7**, 67–74, 1974.

[42] Palmstierna, T. and Wistedt, B. Staff Observation Aggression Scale (SOAS): presentation and evaluation. *Acta Psychiatrica Scand.*, **76**, 657–63, 1987.

[43] Paykel, E.S. Methodological aspects of life event research. *J. Psychosomatic Res.*, **27**, 341–52, 1983.

[44] Peselow, E.D., Filippi, A-M., Goodnick, P., Barouche, F., and Fieve, R.R. The short- and long-term efficacy of paroxetine HCl: A and B. Data from a 6-week double-blind parallel design trial versus imipramine and placebo. *Psychopharmacology Bull.*, **25**, 267–76, 1989.

[45] Rachman, S.J. and Hodgson, R.J. *Obsessions and Compulsions.* Prentice-Hall Inc., Englewood Cliffs, New Jersey, 1980.

[46] Scharfetter, C. (ed). Das AMP-System. Manual zur Dokumentation psychiatrischer Befunde. 2a uppl. Springer-Verlag, Berlin; Heidelberg, New York, 1972.

[47] Simpson, G.M. and Angus, J.W.S. A rating scale for extrapyramidal side effects. *Acta Psychiatrica Scand.*, **46** (Suppl. 212), 11–19, 1979.

[48] Spielberger, C.D., Gorsuch, R.L., and Luschene, R.E. *Manual for the State-Trait Anxiety Inventory.* Consulting Psychologist Press, Palo Alto, 1970.

[49] Taylor, J. The Manifest Anxiety Scale. *J. Abnormal Social Psychol.*, **48**, 285–90, 1953.

[50] Thorén, P., Åsberg, M., Cronholm, B., Jörnestedt, L., and Träskman, L. Clomipramine treatment of obsessive compulsive disorder. I. A controlled clinical trial. *Arch. Gen. Psych.*, **37**, 1281–5, 1980.

[51] van Riezen, H. and Siegel, M. *Comparative Evaluation of Rating Scales for Clinical Psychopharmacology.* Elsevier, Amsterdam, 1988.

[52] Weissman, M.M. The assessment of social adjustment. An update. *Arch. Gen. Psych.*, **38**, 1250–8, 1981.

[53] Wittenborn, J.R. A new procedure for evaluating mental hospital patients. *J. Consulting Psychol.*, **14**, 500–1, 1950.

[54] Young, R.C., Biggs, J.T., Ziegler, V.E., and Meyer, D.A. A rating scale for mania: reliability, validity and sensitivity. *Br. J. Psych.*, **133**, 429–35, 1978.

[55] Yudofsky, S.C., Silver, J.M., Jackson, W., Endicott, J., and Williams, D. The Overt Aggression Scale for the objective rating of verbal and physical aggression. *Am. J. Psych.*, **143**, 35–9, 1986.

[56] Zarifian, E. *Les Jardiniers de la Folie*. Edition Odile Jacob, Paris, p 113, 1988.

[57] Zis, A.P. and Goodwin, F.K. Novel antidepressants and the biogenic amine hypothesis of depression. The case of iprindole and mianserin. *Arch. Gen. Psych.*, **36**, 1097–1107, 1979.

[58] Zung, W.W.K. A self-rating depression scale. *Arch. Gen. Psych.*, **12**, 63–70, 1965.

7. Psychometric Screening of New Drugs

B. Tiplady

Introduction

It is well established that alcohol causes impairment of driving skills and an increase in accidents, and there has been much concern that other drugs might have similar effects.[1,13,37] This has led to increasing use of psychological tests to investigate the effects of drugs on the central nervous system (CNS). For example, tests of reaction time, motor skills and attention may be used to assess drug effects, and thus to support claims concerning the effects of drugs on driving as well as on other everyday activities.[24,31,49]

Attention has been centred on sedative drugs, both those given because of their CNS effects (e.g. hypnotics and anxiolytics) and those for which sedation is an unwanted effect (e.g. antihistamines and antidepressants). Unwanted stimulant effects may also be of concern, as they can lead to sleep problems. Additionally, stimulant effects may indicate a potential for a drug to cause dependence.[70]

Two quite different types of experiment may be distinguished. In the first, the effect under investigation is reasonably well understood, and the purpose is to measure it in a particular situation. For example, with a hypnotic drug given at night, it is of interest to establish whether sedative effects persist the following morning, i.e. does it have a 'hangover effect'?[8,41,54,56] It is important to determine whether sedative drugs have interactions, for example, with alcohol.[27,33,34,48,50] Finally, there may be differences in the magnitude of drug effects in different groups, for example, the young and the elderly.[52,55,57,64] In such studies it is usually straightforward to select appropriate measurements, as the effect in question will be well-documented.

In the second type of study this is not the case. When working with drugs with a new mode of action, the profile of effects on the CNS is naturally unknown. Even a new drug with a familiar mode of action may still have unexpected effects.

This article concentrates on aspects of this screening problem. The principles that should be used in selecting tests for a screening battery are outlined, followed by descriptions of some of the individual tests that are available. Issues of validity are then addressed, and finally the relationship between the magnitude of the effect observed and problems in clinical use are discussed.

The Composition of a Test Battery

Given that we do not know *a priori* what effects a new drug will have, it is important to use a test battery that is as broadly based as possible, i.e. one that samples a wide range of abilities. In order to organise such a selection, some sort of classification of abilities is necessary. A widely accepted approach is to divide abilities into four categories: attention, psychomotor, memory and cognitive.[67] Any battery for screening purposes should include tests under all four of these headings. This represents the *content validity* of the test battery. Other aspects of validity will be considered subsequently.

A second important criterion is that tests should be sensitive to change. Many of the established tests that appear relevant are designed to assess and be stable measures of individual differences. In other words, they are *trait* measures. When investigating drug effects, it is *state* measures, those capable of detecting change within an individual, that are required.

This presents a particular problem when studying potentially novel drug actions, as it is not adequate simply to use tests that are known to detect familiar drug effects such as sedation. A new drug may affect behaviour in quite different ways from a sedative. Thus other types of effect may be used as indicators of the sensitivity of a test to change within an individual. When selecting potential tests from the literature, we have used such factors as ageing and sleep deprivation, as well as the effects of several classes of drug, as indicators of sensitivity to change.

Tests must, of course, be reliable. However, it is important to note that the criteria for reliability are not the same as those used in most branches of psychometrics. Measures such as the test-retest reliability are appropriate for trait measures. With state measures, a test-retest measure would be appropriate only if we could ensure that the state of the individual was constant on the two occasions, which is not generally the case. Much more useful is a within-test measure, such as the split-half reliability. However, this also has its limitations, being the ratio of the variability of the test to the variability of the population. Thus, a relatively homogeneous population will lead to a low measured reliability, but this will not preclude sensitivity to drug effects within that population.

A final requirement is that tests be suitable for repeated use. Most psychometric studies will follow a drug effect over several hours. Many are crossover studies with three or four periods. It is quite common for a particular test to be administered more than 20 times in one study. Some tests lend themselves readily to such use, since the test material is automatically generated for each trial. This is the case, for example, with reaction time tests. In other cases, multiple sets of test material must be generated, and shown to be equivalent.

To illustrate the variety of measures that are available, some commonly used tests will now be described. This selection is by no means exhaustive, but will give examples of tests in all of the main categories listed above.

Measures of Attention

The most commonly used attention tasks are of vigilance, concentrated attention and divided attention.

Vigilance

Tests of vigilance are characterised by the detection of signals which are small, often close to the threshold of detection, over substantial periods. An example is the Wilkinson Auditory Vigilance Task.[69] In this test, the subject listens through headphones to a series of tones against a background of white noise. Most of the tones are 500 msec long, but an occasional tone is 400 msec. The subject's task is to press a button each time a short tone is heard. The test typically lasts one hour.

This is a difficult test, the average performance being approximately 50% of correct detections. The test is sensitive, being able to detect the effects of relatively low doses of sedative drugs, and also of mild stimulants such as caffeine and theophylline.[9,19,23,61] The usefulness of the test is limited by its duration, as it is clearly not possible to follow the time-course of action of a drug with any precision using a one-hour measure.

Concentrated Attention

A suitable test of this is the Continuous Performance Test.[45] In this test, a series of different letters is flashed on a screen and the subject has to respond each time an X (easy condition) or an X preceded by an A (hard condition) is seen. The interval between letters is 0.92 sec, and the test lasts either 5 or 10 min. The test is capable of detecting the effects of brain damage (for which it was originally developed), sleep deprivation and drugs such as barbiturates and chlorpromazine, the latter having a particularly marked effect.[35]

An alternative test is the Continuous Attention Task.[59] This uses geometric patterns as stimuli (*Figure 7.1*), the subject's task being to respond whenever two consecutive shapes are the same. The intervals between stimuli are randomised (1.5–2.5 sec) and the test lasts about 8 min. The use of non-verbal material may be an advantage, and the randomisation of the intervals ensures the need for attention to be sustained rather than paced to the regular rhythm of stimulus presentation. The test is sensitive to the effects of a number of drugs, including mianserin, chlormethiazole, nitrous oxide and, in the elderly, caffeine.[16,17,56,57]

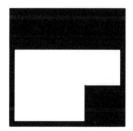 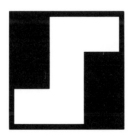 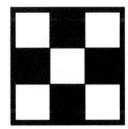

Figure 7.1. A selection of figures from the Continuous Attention Task. The subject should respond whenever two consecutive patterns are the same. Patterns are shown with black and white reversed, as they are displayed on a dark screen.

Divided Attention

Measures of divided attention may be more sensitive to the effects of some drugs, in particular alcohol. The usual paradigm is to use a central task, such as tracking, coupled with a peripheral signal detection task.[38,39]

Psychomotor Tests

A great variety of psychomotor tests, both automated and using paper and pencil, is available.

Pencil-and-Paper Tests
Two commonly used tests are the Gibson Spiral Maze and the Digit–Symbol Substitution Test. In the Spiral Maze[21], the subject follows a spiral path marked on a sheet of paper while attempting to avoid the sides of the path and a series of obstacles. The time taken and the number of errors are recorded. In the substitution test[51,66], there is a key in which the numbers 1–9 are each matched to a symbol. A series of random numbers is printed on a grid on the sheet and subjects write the corresponding symbol under each digit as quickly as possible. The number of correct and incorrect symbols written in a fixed time, often 90 sec, is recorded. Automated versions of the Digit–Symbol test have been used by a number of groups.[25,32,72]

Psychomotor Speed
A commonly used test of psychomotor speed is the Choice Reaction Time, such as that incorporated in the Leeds Psychomotor Tester.[20] The apparatus has six buttons arranged in a semicircle, by each of which is a light. A seventh button is located at the centre. The subject places the index finger on the central button. At varying intervals, one or other of the lights comes on, whereupon the subject moves his finger to touch the corresponding button as quickly as possible. The latency (time to move the finger from the start button) and total reaction time are measured, and movement time is obtained by subtraction. This test is capable of detecting the effects of a wide range of CNS depressant drugs, including benzodiazepines, barbiturates and antidepressants.[26,28]

Critical Flicker Fusion Threshold
This is not strictly speaking a psychomotor test, and may rather be considered as an index of central processing speed. It is included here because it is probably more closely related to this group of tests than to any other. The test establishes the minimum frequency at which a flickering light appears steady (fusion) or the maximum frequency at which flicker can be detected. This threshold frequency is generally lowered by sedative drugs.[26]

Saccadic Eye Movements
Eye movements are of two kinds – slow pursuit movements, and rapid saccadic movements. Their measurement requires specialised equipment, but is straightforward for the subject. The peak velocity and accuracy of saccades are reduced by several CNS depressant drugs, including benzodiazepines, alcohol and barbiturates.[3,22,30] Saccadic eye movements are of particular interest in that, once initiated, they are largely independent of voluntary control, and thus are relatively little affected by the level of attention.

Body Sway

This is a measure of psychomotor coordination rather than speed. One simple apparatus consists of a box with a string.[71] The box is placed at a height of 1 m above the ground, and the string is attached to the standing subject at the same height. The apparatus sums the movements in the anterior–posterior plane over a one-minute period, giving a measure of body sway. It can demonstrate the effects of a wide range of sedative drugs.[53]

Tracking

Tests of tracking are commonly used, at least partly because of their similarity to one component of driving. Some tasks use a joystick similar to that employed in computer games, some use a steering wheel in various degrees of driving simulation, and in some cases actual driving is used.[6,10,28,40,65]

Tests of Memory

The tests available may be divided into verbal and non-verbal, and into those of short-term and long-term memory.

Selective Reminding

This verbal memory test gives an assessment of aspects of both long- and short-term memory.[7] A list of words is read to the subject at 2 sec intervals. The subject tries to recall the words in any order (free recall). The subject is then reminded only of those words that were not recalled correctly, and then attempts again to recall all the words in the list. This procedure is repeated until the list is completely recalled. Items recalled on a recall attempt that were not reminded before that attempt are considered to have been retrieved from long-term memory. The test thus allows the separation of retrieval from long- and short-term storage, and can also separate consistent and inconsistent long-term recall. This test has been used in a number of studies where memory has been of interest, in particular with anticholinergic drugs.[5,43,44]

Paired Word Learning

This is a simpler test that does not distinguish between short- and long-term memory.[29] The subject is presented with three word pairs, following which the first word of the pair is given as a cue. The subject responds by saying the second. This is repeated until each cue word has been presented three times. The procedure is then repeated with two further sets of three word pairs (*Figure 7.2*). The test shows memory impairments with benzodiazepines and other sedative drugs, including chlormethiazole and nitrous oxide.[16,17]

Spatial Learning

A test analogous to the Verbal Selective Reminding Test has been developed which uses pairs of rectangles from an irregular grid instead of words. This has been shown to detect the effects of scopolamine.[43]

Cognitive Tests

The tests in this category form a rather heterogeneous group, ranging from slightly elaborated tests of attention to tests that explore quite deep levels of processing.

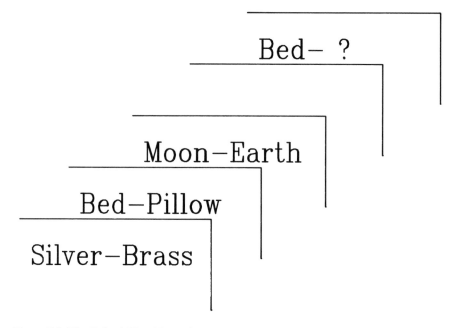

Figure 7.2. The Paired-Word Learning Test. Three word pairs are displayed on a monitor screen for 3 sec each. The subject is then presented with the first word of a pair, and should respond by saying the second, in this case 'pillow'. Each cue word is presented three times in random order.

Rapid Information Processing
The subject is presented with a sequence of digits at a rate typically of 100/min. Presentation may be either aural[58] or on a monitor screen.[68] The task is to respond either to three successive even digits or to three successive odd digits. The test has been shown to detect impairments due to scopolamine, as well as improvements with nicotine.[68]

Arithmetic
Many studies have used some sort of test of arithmetic.[14,15] A test as simple as subtracting 7 from 100 repeatedly is sufficient to detect ethanol impairment.[15]

Semantic Processing
Subjects are presented with a series of sentences. Some are true, e.g. 'Horses have legs'. Others are false, e.g. 'Bicycles have wings'. The subject presses a *yes* or *no* button as quickly as possible to indicate whether the sentence is true or not. The test has been shown to be capable of detecting ethanol impairments.[2]

Subjective Measures
Assessment of subjective awareness of drug effects is important for two reasons. Firstly, the effects of drugs may be experienced as unpleasant by the subject, and this needs to be documented as it may affect compliance.

Secondly, under some circumstances subjective measures may be more sensitive than objective tests, or may pick up effects that are beyond the scope of the test battery.[19] The most commonly used subjective measure is the Visual Analogue Scale, which consists of a 100 mm line marked at each end with semantic opposites, e.g. 'alert–drowsy', or 'interested–bored'. The subject makes a mark on the line to indicate his or her feelings at the time. The position of the mark on the scale is measured in millimetres.[4]

Hierarchical Organisation

In considering the types of tests described above, it is clear that in several cases the abilities being tested may be arranged in hierarchical fashion. Thus, any test with a speeded response, such as the Sentence Verification Test, will depend on psychomotor speed. Any test of memory will depend on attention. This is illustrated in *Figure 7.3*. In general, any impairment at a low level in the hierarchy will be reflected in reduced performance on the higher level tests, whether or not the higher level ability is actually impaired. This must always be borne in mind in the interpretation of study results, and to this end it is important that the lower level tests should always be included in the battery.

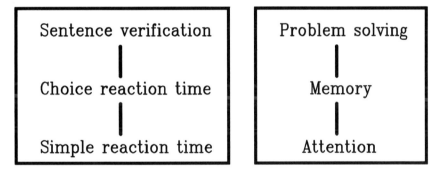

Figure 7.3. Psychometric hierarchies: a test of higher-level ability will involve lower-level abilities also. Thus, if attention is impaired, reduced performance on a memory test may be expected even if no actual impairment of memory mechanisms is present.

Construct Validity

If studies are to be interpreted in a meaningful way, the measures used must be valid, i.e. they must measure what they purport to measure. A number of different forms of validation may be distinguished, namely construct, content, concurrent, criterion and face validity. Content validity has been dealt with above, and in the present context usually refers to the scope of a test *battery*, rather than the content of an individual test. Construct validity concerns the extent to which the test measures some theoretical construct. Examples of constructs that may be of interest are arousal, attention, short-term memory and long-term memory. A test, for example, that was intended to assess arousal level would be expected to show decrements following sleep deprivation or during prolonged task performance.

In many cases such validity may be inferred from the way the test is set up and the nature of the constructs. Thus, in the Selective Reminding Test[7], the involvement of long-term memory in items recalled correctly on the second list recall, that were not reminded on the first, can be derived simply from the time-scale of forgetting from the short-term store. If the constructs of long- and short-term memory are appropriate, the short-term store cannot be involved, and so the long-term store must be. Note that the reverse cannot be said. The involvement of the long-term store in items recalled shortly after presentation cannot be ruled out in this way.

Such argument by elimination is often necessary, for a valid test must not only be influenced by the things it should be measuring, but should not be influenced by other factors. Thus, a test of attention should not be affected by memory limitations, and a test of memory should not be affected by differences in comprehension of material. It is for this reason that memory tests generally use either nonsense material (which will be understood by none of the subjects) or common words (that will be understood by all subjects). It should be noted that, where abilities are arranged hierarchically, test results may be affected by factors lower on the hierarchy (which usually cannot be avoided), but should not be affected by those at a higher level.

Separate experiments may be needed to establish that tests are not being affected by irrelevant factors, a procedure known as discriminant validation. Using such a procedure, for example, the Continuous Attention Task has been shown not to be limited by the rate of transfer of information from perceptual memory into the short-term store, nor by the capacity of the short-term store.

Criterion Validity

This is a form of validity of particular importance in practical terms. It concerns the ability of the test to predict outcome on some external measure, accidents being the outcome of most general concern. Rather few of the tests in use have been adequately validated in this way, and indeed it is a very difficult task to do so except to a very limited extent.

Body Sway
One such limited, but valuable, study concerns the use of body sway as a correlate of falls in the elderly. Overstall et al.[42] measured body sway using the apparatus described above[71], and also took a history of falls in a group of 243 elderly subjects and in a control group of 63 younger people. They found a significant correlation between sway in the elderly and the incidence of falls, and also between body sway and age. Clearly this can only be taken as evidence of validity in the elderly – the incidence of falls in the young is far too small for any generalisation to be useful. However, it is in the elderly that there is particular concern about the use of sedatives (which have marked effects on sway), in terms of both frequency of use and the possibility of longer action or greater sensitivity to drug effects.

Sleepiness on the job
In a study of drivers of electric locomotives in Sweden, Torsvall and Akerstedt[62] observed 11 drivers over a period of 4.5 h, during journeys both at night and during the day. They measured EEG, as well as ECG and EOG. In some subjects the EEG showed episodic changes, consisting of an increase in alpha and theta rhythms. These changes correlated with performance lapses as well as with reported and observed sleepiness. This finding indicates the importance of correlating EEG changes with performance on attention tasks.[11,24,63]

The examples given above may be also taken as evidence of *ecological validity*, since the outcome measures and abilities in question are clearly relevant to the subject's normal life.

Face Validity

Some measures appear by their format to be particularly relevant to real-life situations, for example, tests involving driving simulation or actual driving.[28,40,65] In some situations, simulations are clearly valid, as, for example, the simulation of a radar screen for watch-keeping or air traffic control tasks, where the simulated display and the performance measured may be essentially identical to the real thing. A completely realistic assessment of driving, however, would require assessment of many thousands of hours of performance for each accident, near-miss or serious error of judgement, which is clearly not practicable. What are used in such circumstances are measures of performance such as tracking, reaction time or divided attention, assessed in as naturalistic a fashion as possible. The most realistic is of course actual driving. For example, O'Hanlon and co-workers use the standard deviation of lateral position (SDLP) during 100 km of real driving as an index of performance.[40] This is a measure analogous to the root mean square deviation generally used in laboratory tracking tasks.

Such a measure clearly *looks* more valid (face validity) than, say, a laboratory-based tracking task using a joystick, but it is not possible to be sure that it is so. Firstly, it is not self-evident that an increase in SDLP is in fact associated with an increase in accidents, which is what actually matters. Many factors are involved in driving skill, including attention, tracking ability, reaction time and risk perception. The relative importance of these factors is not obvious, neither is the best method of assessing them. It may well be that a laboratory-based test is a more sensitive indicator than a real-life driving test. Equally tracking, unless grossly impaired, might have little to do with accidents. It is precisely the function of a validation study to determine this. It is interesting in this context that alcohol, known to have a major effect on traffic accidents from epidemiological data, has relatively little effect on simple psychomotor tasks, while having substantial effects on tests involving either divided attention or a cognitive component.[38,39,60] This suggests that it may be such skills that are more important for drug-induced impairments causing accidents. This again indicates the importance of assessing a broad range of abilities, rather than just a single aspect of behaviour.

Magnitude of Effects

Even if our tests are valid, appropriate and reliable, there still remains the question of how to interpret an effect of a particular size. What does a slowing of 100 msec or a decrease in flicker fusion frequency of 2 Hz mean in terms of everyday life? A slowing of 100 msec is equivalent to about 3 m additional stopping distance when driving at 110 km/h (approximately 70 m.p.h.), an increase of 3–4% on the normal stopping distance.[12] Even this does not really help much in assessing any increase in accident risk.

Ideally, if criterion validation data were available in sufficient detail, it would be possible to establish a direct numerical relation between the various types of impairment and increased risk. Since this is not available, the best that can be done is, firstly, to assess the profiles of drugs so that areas of particular concern can be identified and given further study; and, secondly, where profiles are similar, to assess the relative impairments by different drugs.

This may be illustrated by a comparison of two recent studies carried out by our group on drugs with quite different actions.[16,18] One, chlormethiazole, is a sedative/hypnotic. The second, remoxipride, is a dopamine-2 receptor antagonist which is under development as an antipsychotic. Each has been investigated in healthy volunteers in order to assess sedative and other psychometric effects, and the results of these studies are summarised in *Table 7.1.* It is clear, first of all, that chlormethiazole produced impairments on all measures assessed. Such a global pattern represents a typical sedative profile, and is similar to that seen with benzodiazepines or antihistamines. The pattern with remoxipride was quite different. Remoxipride had much less sedative effect than chlormethiazole, as indicated by the subjective 'alert–drowsy' rating. It also had less effect on choice reaction latency, little or no effect on body sway and, if anything, improved the motor component of choice reaction time. However, remoxipride had a larger effect on continuous attention, corresponding to a near doubling of the error rate compared to chlormethiazole. This kind of double-dissociation is important, for it shows that the differences in profile are not merely due to the use of non-equivalent doses.

Table 7.1. A comparison of the maximum effects* of chlormethiazole and remoxipride on some measures of CNS function.

	Remoxipride	Chlormethiazole
Alert–drowsy VAS (mm)	+19	+52
CAT total errors	+ 7.0	+ 3.9
CRT latency (msec)	+42	+75
CRT movement time (msec)	−31	+26
Sway (degrees/3)	(1)[†]	+ 7.9
Time to peak effect (h)	4–6	0–1

* Maximum effect (active *minus* placebo) at any time point was taken for 447 mg chlormethiazole[16] and for 60 mg remoxipride[18] in young volunteers. Abbreviations: VAS, Visual Analogue Scale (100 mm); CAT, Continuous Attention Task; CRT, Choice Reaction Time.
† Neither a clear increase nor a clear decrease with drug compared to placebo.

The difference between remoxipride and the more typical sedative profile of chlormethiazole is not entirely unexpected, as other neuroleptic drugs have shown comparable effects. Thus, Mirsky and Rosvold[36] showed a double-dissociation between barbiturates and chlorpromazine, the former having a relatively greater effect on a psychomotor task (Digit–Symbol Substitution) while the latter showed more effect on an attention task (the Continuous Performance Task). Selective effects of haloperidol on attention have also been reported.[46,47] This may, therefore, represent a characteristic profile of neuroleptic agents.

Conclusions

A wide range of psychometric measures is available for assessment of the effects of drugs on various aspects of CNS function. Much remains to be done in clarifying the relationship between changes in test performance and everyday activities. However, test results are of great value in making comparisons between drugs, and in providing a profile of CNS effects.

References

[1] Altmann, P., Hamon, C., Blair, J., Dhanesha, U., Cunningham, J., and Marsh, F. Disturbance of cerebral function by aluminium in haemodialysis patients without overt aluminium toxicity. *Lancet*, ii, 7–12, 1989.

[2] Baddeley, A.D. The cognitive psychology of everyday life. *Br. J. Psychol.*, 72, 257–69, 1981.

[3] Bittencourt, P.R.M. *et al.* The relationship between peak velocity of saccadic eye movements and serum benzodiazepine concentrations. *Br. J. Clin. Pharmacol.*, 12, 523–33, 1981.

[4] Bond, A. and Lader, M. The use of analogue scales in rating subjective feelings. *Br. J. Med. Psychol.*, 47, 211–18, 1974.

[5] Branconnier, R.J., Devitt, D.R., Cole, J.O. and Spera, K.F. Amitriptyline selectively disrupts verbal recall from secondary memory of the normal aged. *Neurobiol. Ageing*, 3, 55–9, 1982.

[6] Burns, M. and Moskowitz, H. Effects of diphenhydramine and alcohol on skills performance. *Eur. J. Clin. Pharmacol.*, 17, 259–66, 1980.

[7] Buschke, H. and Fuld, P.A. Evaluating storage, retention and retrieval in disordered memory and learning. *Neurology*, 24, 1019–25, 1974.

[8] Clarke, C.H. and Nicholson, A.N. Immediate and residual effects in man of the metabolites of diazepam. *Br. J. Clin. Pharmacol.*, 6, 325–31, 1978.

[9] Clubley, M., Bye, C.E., Henson, T.A., Peck, A.W., and Riddington, C.J. Effects of caffeine and cyclizine alone and in combination on human performance, subjective effects and EEG activity. *Br. J. Clin. Pharmacol.*, 7, 157–63, 1979.

[10] Cohen, A.F., Ashby, L., Crowley, D., Land, G., Peck, A.W., and Miller, A.A. Lamotrigine (BW430C), a potential anticonvulsant. Effects on the central nervous system in comparison with phenytoin and diazepam. *Br. J. Clin. Pharmacol.*, 20, 619–29, 1985.

[11] Davies, D.R. and Parasuraman, R. *The Psychology of Vigilance.* Academic Press, London, pp 180–207, 1982.

[12] Dept. of Transport, Central Office of Information. *The Highway Code.* HMSO, London, p 14, 1987.

[13] Donelson, A.C., Monks, M.E., Jones, R.K., and Joscelyn, K.B. *The alcohol-highway safety experience and its applicability to other drugs.* National Highway Safety Administration, DOT-HS-805 374, 1980.

[14] Ekman, G., Frankenhauser, M., Goldberg, L., Bjerver, K., Jarpe, G., and Myrsten, A-L. Effects of alcohol intake on subjective and objective variables over a five-hour period. *Psychopharmacologia*, **4**, 28–38, 1963.

[15] Evans, M.A., Martz, R., Rodda, B.E. *et al.* Quantitative relationship between blood alcohol concentration and psychomotor performance. *Clin. Pharmacol. Therapeutics*, 253–60, 1973.

[16] Fagan, D., Lamont, M., Jostell, K-G., Tiplady, B., and Scott, D.B. A study of the psychometric effects of chlormethiazole in healthy young and elderly subjects. *Age and Ageing* (in press).

[17] Fagan, D., Paul, D., Drummond, G., Scott, D.B., and Tiplady, B. A dose-response study of the effects of nitrous oxide on mood and performance in healthy volunteers. Abstracts of the Meeting of the British Association for Psychopharmacology, Cambridge, July 1989. *J. Psychopharmacol.*, **3**, 98, 1989.

[18] Fagan, D., Scott, D.B., and Mitchell, M. The psychomotor effects of remoxipride in healthy volunteers. *Neuroscience Lett.*, S32; S45, 1988.

[19] Fagan, D., Swift, C.G., and Tiplady, B. Effects of caffeine on vigilance and other performance tests in normal subjects. *J. Psychopharmacol.*, **2**, 19–25, 1988.

[20] Frewer, L.J. and Hindmarch, I. The effects of time of day, age and anxiety on a choice reaction task. In *Psychopharmacology and Reaction Time*, I. Hindmarch, B. Aufdembrinke, and H. Ott (eds), Wiley, Chichester, pp 103–14, 1988.

[21] Gibson, H.B. *Manual to the Gibson Spiral Maze.* 2nd edition, Hodder and Stoughton Educational, Sevenoaks, Kent, 1978.

[22] Griffiths, A.N., Marshall, R.W., and Richens, A. Saccadic eye movement analysis as a measure of drug effects on human psychomotor performance. *Br. J. Clin. Pharmacol.*, **18**, 73S–83S, 1984.

[23] Hart, J., Hill, H.M., Bye, C.E., Wilkinson, R.T., and Peck, A.W. The effects of low doses of amylobarbitone sodium and diazepam on human performance. *Br. J. Clin. Pharmacol.*, **3**, 289–98, 1976.

[24] Herrman, W.M. and Baumgartner, P. Combined pharmaco-EEG and pharmacopsychological study to estimate CNS effects of ketanserin in hypertensive patients. *Neuropsychobiology*, **16**, 47–56, 1986.

[25] Higgins, S.T., Lamb, R.J., and Henningfield, J.E. Dose-dependent effects of atropine on behavioural and physiologic responses in humans. *Pharmacol. Biochem. Behav.*, **34**, 303–11, 1989.

[26] Hindmarch, I. Psychomotor function and psychoactive drugs. *Br. J. Pharmac.*, **10**, 189–209, 1980.

[27] Hindmarch, I. and Subhan, Z. The effects of antidepressants taken with and without alcohol on information processing, psychomotor performance and car handling ability. In *Drugs and Driving*, J.F. O'Hanlon and J.J. de Gier (eds), Taylor & Francis, London, 1986.

[28] Hindmarch, I., Subhan, Z., and Stoker, M. The effects of zimeldine and amitriptyline on car driving and psychomotor performance. *Acta Psychiatr. Scand.*, **28** (Suppl. 308), 141, 1983.

[29] Isaacs, B. and Walkey, F.A. A simplified paired-associate test for elderly hospital patients. *Br. J. Psychiat.*, **110**, 80–3, 1964.

[30] King, D.J. and Bell, P. The effect of temazepam on psychomotor performance and saccadic eye movements. Abstracts of the meeting of the British Association for Psychopharmacology, Cambridge, July 1988. *J. Psychopharmacol.*, **2**(2), 1988.

[31] Laurell, H. and Tournros, J. The carry-over effects of triazolam compared with nitrazepam and placebo in acute emergency driving situations and in monotonous simulated driving. *Acta Pharmacol. Toxicol.*, **58**, 182–6, 1986.

[32] Lex, B.W., Lukas, S.E., Greenwald, N.E., and Mendelson, J.H. Alcohol-induced changes in women at risk from alcoholism. *J. Stud. Alcohol*, **49**, 346–56, 1988.

[33] Linnoila, M., Mattila, M.J., and Kitchell, B.S. Drug interactions with alcohol. *Drugs*, **18**, 299–311, 1979.

[34] Milner, G. Amitriptyline – potentiation of alcohol. *Lancet*, 222–3, 28 January 1967.

[35] Mirsky, A.F. and Kornetsky, C. On the dissimilar effects of drugs on the digit symbol substitution and continuous performance tests. *Psychopharmacologia*, **5**, 161–77, 1964.

[36] Mirsky, A.F. and Rosvold, H.E. The use of psychoactive drugs as a neuropsychological tool in studies of attention in man. In *Drugs and Behavior*, L. Uhr and J.G. Miller (eds), 375–92, 1960.

[37] Mortimer, R.G. and Howat, P.A. Effects of alcohol and diazepam, singly and in combination, on some aspects of driving performance. In *Drugs and Driving*, J.F. O'Hanlon and J.J. de Gier (eds), Taylor & Francis, London, 1986.

[38] Moskowitz, H. Attention tasks as skills performance measures of drug effects. *Br. J. Clin. Pharmacol.*, **18**, 51S–61S, 1984.

[39] Moskowitz, H. and Sharma, S. Effects of alcohol on peripheral vision as a function of attention. *Human Factors*, **16**, 174–80, 1974.

[40] O'Hanlon, J.F. Driving performance under the influence of drugs: rationale for, and application of, a new test. *Br. J. Clin. Pharmacol.*, **18**, 121S–129S, 1984.

[41] Ogura, C., Nakazawa, K., Majima, K. *et al.* Residual effects of hypnotics: triazolam, flurazepam and nitrazepam. *Psychopharmacol.*, **68**, 61–5, 1980.

[42] Overstall, W., Exton-Smith, A.N., Imms, F.J., and Johnson, A.L. Falls in the elderly related to postural imbalance. *Br. Med. J.*, **1**, 261–4, 1977.

[43] Preston, G.C., Brazell, C., Ward, C., Broks, P., Traub, M., and Stahl, S.M. The scopolamine model of dementia: determination of central choinomimetic effects of physostigmine on cognition and biochemical markers in man. *J. Psychopharmacol.* **2**, 67–79, 1988.

[44] Preston, G.C., Ward, C., Lines, C.R., Poppleton, P., Haigh, J.R.M., and Traub, M. Scopolamine and benzodiazepine models of dementia: cross-reversals by Ro 15–1788 and physostigmine. *Psychopharmacol.*, **98**, 487–94, 1989.

[45] Rosvold, H.E., Mirsky, A.F., Sarason, I., Bransome, E.D., Jr, and Beck, L.H. A continuous performance test of brain damage. *J. Consulting Psychology*, **20**, 343–50, 1956.

[46] Saletu, B., Grunberger, J., Linzmayer, L., and Dubini, A. Determinations of pharmacodynamics of the new neuroleptic zetidoline by neuroendocrinolo-

gic, pharmaco-EEG, and psychometric studies – Part I. *Internat. J. Clin. Pharm. Ther. Tox.*, **21**, 489–95, 1983.

[47] Saletu, B., Grunberger, J., Linzmayer, L., and Dubini, A. Determination of the pharmacodynamics of the new neuroleptic zetidoline by neuroendocrinologic, pharmaco-EEG, and psychometric studies – Part II. *Internat. J. Clin. Pharm. Ther. Tox.*, **21**, 544–51, 1983.

[48] Scott, D.B., Fagan, D., and Tiplady, B. Effects of amitriptyline and zimelidine in combination with ethanol. *Psychopharmacol.*, **76**, 209–11, 1982.

[49] Smiley, A. and Moskowitz, H. Effects of long-term administration of buspirone and diazepam on driver steering control. *Am. J. Med.*, **80**, 22–9, 1986.

[50] Starmer, G.A. and Bird, K.D. Investigating drug-ethanol interactions. *Br. J. Clin. Pharmacol.*, **18**, 27S–35S, 1984.

[51] Stone, B.M. Pencil and paper tests – sensitivity to psychotropic drugs. *Br. J. Clin. Pharmacol.*, **18**, 15S–20S, 1984.

[52] Swift, C.G. *Studies on the Response to Benzodiazepines in the Elderly*, PhD Thesis, University of Dundee, 1983.

[53] Swift, C.G. Postural instability as a measure of sedative drug response. *Br. J. Clin. Pharmacol.*, **18**, 87S–90S, 1984.

[54] Swift, C.G., Ewen, J.N., Clarke, P., and Stevenson, I.H. Responsiveness to oral diazepam in the elderly: relationship to total and free plasma concentrations. *Br. J. Clin. Pharmacol.*, **20**, 111–18, 1985.

[55] Swift, C.G., Haythorne, J.M., Clarke, P., and Stevenson, I.H. The effect of ageing on measured responses to single doses of oral temazepam. *Br. J. Clin. Pharmacol.*, **11**, 413P–414P, 1980.

[56] Swift, C.G., Swift, M.R., and Tiplady, B. 'First-dose' response to mianserin: effects of age. *Psychopharmacol.*, **96**, 273–6, 1988.

[57] Swift, C.G. and Tiplady, B. The effects of age on the response to caffeine. *Psychopharmacol.*, **94**, 29–31, 1988.

[58] Talland, G.A. Effects of alcohol on performance in continuous attention tasks. *Psychosom. Med.*, **28**, 596–604, 1966.

[59] Tiplady, B. A continuous attention test for the assessment of the acute behavioural effects of drugs. *Psychopharmacol. Bull.*, **24**, 213–16, 1988.

[60] Tiplady, B. Alcohol as a comparator. In *Ambulatory Anaesthesia and Sedation*, I.D. Klepper, L.D. Sanders, and M. Rosen (eds), Blackwells, Oxford, pp 26–37, 1991.

[61] Tiplady, B., Fagan, D., Lamont, M., Brockway, M., and Scott, D.B. A comparison of the CNS effects of enprofylline and theophylline in healthy subjects assessed by performance testing and subjective measures. *Br. J. Clin. Pharmacol.*, **30**, 55–61, 1990.

[62] Torsvall, L. and Akerstedt, T. Sleepiness on the job: continuously measured EEG changes in train drivers. *Electroenceph. Clin. Neurophysiol.*, **66**, 502–11, 1987.

[63] Valley, V. and Broughton, R. The physiological (EEG) nature of drowsiness and its relation to performance deficits in narcoleptics. *Electroenceph. Clin. Neurophysiol.*, **55**, 243–51, 1983.

[64] Veith, R.C. Treatment of psychiatric disorders. In *Drug Treatment in the Elderly*, R.E. Vestal (ed), ADIS, Sydney, 1984.

[65] Volkerts, E.R. and O'Hanlon, J.F. Hypnotics' residual effects on driving performance. In *Drugs and Driving*, J.F. O'Hanlon and J.J. de Gier (eds), Taylor & Francis, London, 1986.

[66] Wechsler, D. *The measurement and appraisal of human intelligence*, 4th edition, Williams & Wilkins, Baltimore, 1958.

[67] Wesnes, K., Simpson P., and Christmas, L. The assessment of human information-processing abilities in psychopharmacology. In *Human Psychopharmacology*, Methods and Measures Vol. I, I. Hindmarch and P.D. Stonier (eds), Wiley, Chichester, 1987.

[68] Wesnes, K. and Warburton, D.M. Effects of smoking on rapid visual information processing performance. *Neuropsychobiol.*, **9**, 223–9, 1983.

[69] Wilkinson, R.T. Sleep deprivation: performance tests for partial and selective sleep deprivation. *Prog. Clin. Psychol.*, **8**, 28–43, 1968.

[70] Wise, R.A. The role of reward pathways in the development of drug dependence. *Pharmacol. Ther.*, **35**, 227–63, 1987.

[71] Wright, B.M. A simple mechanical ataxiameter. *J. Physiol.*, **218**, 27P–28P, 1971.

[72] Yu, G., Maskrey, V., Jackson, S.H.D., Tiplady, B., and Swift, C.G.S. A comparison of the CNS effects of caffeine and theophylline in elderly subjects. *Br. J. Clin. Pharm.* (in press).

8. Pain Models in Healthy Volunteers

J. Posner

Why Pain Models?

Evaluation of the relationship between dose or plasma concentration and response in man is essential for optimising the design of clinical trials of new drugs. Although the effect must be assessed ultimately in patients, early studies in healthy volunteers can contribute enormously to drug development. Measurement of pharmacodynamic variables, including adverse effects, can be combined with pharmacokinetic data in the relevant dose range. On the basis of such information, recommendations may be made about dosage and predictions made about the likely therapeutic index.

There are numerous validated and objective non-invasive techniques which can be used to measure the activity of drugs affecting the cardiovascular and respiratory systems. Many of these are quite simple. Thus the effective dose of a beta-blocking drug can be ascertained by measuring exercise heart rate, that of a bronchodilator may be assessed by measuring forced expiratory volume (FEV_1) after bronchial challenge, and the dose-range of an angiotensin-converting enzyme (ACE) inhibitor can be defined on the basis of assay of the enzyme in plasma. In contrast, assessment of analgesic activity is not straightforward, for pain is a complex sensation which defies objective measurement. 'Pain' has been defined by the International Association for the Study of Pain as 'an unpleasant sensory and emotional experience associated with actual or potential tissue damage or described in terms of such damage'. It involves a stimulus, nociception and sensation, and also components of suffering and behaviour. Any attempt to measure pain under laboratory conditions must inevitably eliminate much of the reactive component and the element of surprise which is important in many traumatic situations.

Given the artificial conditions in the laboratory and the difficulty in obtaining measurements of this subjective phenomenon, it is not surprising that the view has often been expressed that there is no place for studies of experimental pain.[1,32] Furthermore, until fairly recently, those who did venture into the minefield of laboratory testing of analgesics in man usually concentrated on the 'pain threshold', which is probably the least susceptible component of pain sensation to the action of analgesics. The much-cited paper of Wolff, Hardy and Goodell published in 1941[69], in which they claimed that aspirin and other analgesics elevated the pain threshold to radiant heat, generated a great deal of enthusiasm for experimental analge-simetry, but few other workers were able to reproduce their results. Beecher[1] concluded that the pain threshold was not only a highly variable and impure perception, but also that it was unresponsive to the action of powerful analgesics. He considered the pain threshold in man, in contrast to that of animals, to be a value judgement of the cortex and unsuitable for the study of analgesics. He was probably correct, but, as his own work subsequently showed, analgesic effects in man can be demonstrated in the laboratory by assessing modalities other than pain threshold. Such experiments cannot substitute for clinical trials in patients suffering from headache, post-operative or chronic pain, but in this respect pain models are no different from other pharmacological models. Measurements of heart rate, FEV_1 or ACE activity are no less surrogates for angina pectoris, asthma or cardiac failure. From the point of view of the clinical pharmacologist, they are all valid if quantification of the relationship between dose and effect can be used to make reasonably accurate predictions of the dosage requirements and efficacy of a drug in the clinical situation.

Providing pain models do indeed have predictive value, their potential advantages are worthy of consideration. Unlike clinical trials in patients, the experimental pain model enables a reproducible stimulus of quantifiable intensity to be applied in a carefully controlled environment. The effect of various doses may be examined in a much shorter time than in clinical trials, using a small number of subjects trained to rate pain intensity in response to such a known stimulus. Results are not confounded by concomitant medication or disease or variation in the painful condition itself. The relationships between plasma concentration and effect, duration of action and associated effects may thus be defined.

Owing to the subjective nature of the measurements, the design and conduct of studies must be meticulous. Single-dose studies will usually be of a crossover design with the order of treatments randomised and balanced, and administered under double-blind conditions. As well as placebo, a standard dose of an established analgesic should be used as a positive control both to provide a check on the model, thereby avoiding misinterpretation of false negative results with the drug under test, and to estimate the dosage equivalence.

The Pain Model

Criteria

For an experimental pain model to be acceptable and valid, it must have certain characteristics:

- The stimulus must not cause significant tissue damage.
- The stimulus must be quantifiable so that it can be administered on repeated occasions in a highly reproducible manner.
- The stimulus must cause a sensation that is unequivocally identified by the subject as painful, and it should be possible to adjust the stimulus strength to produce a perceptible range of pain intensity ranging from slight to severe.

- The pain response must be quantifiable and it must be specifically suppressed by analgesics, i.e. sedatives and other drugs which do not exhibit analgesic properties in the clinical situation should not be effective.
- The model should be sufficiently sensitive for the effect of analgesics to be demonstrable using normal therapeutic doses in small groups of volunteers who may be considered representative of the general population.

The Stimulus

A great number of different painful stimuli have been tried with varying degrees of success, often reflecting the care with which physical principles have been considered and test conditions controlled. The stimuli may be classified generically into thermal, electrical, chemical, mechanical and ischaemic (*Table 8.1*).

These techniques have been the subject of reviews[3,44,53] and not all are described fully here, as disappointingly few have been tested rigorously with analgesics. Instead, just two of these techniques (the ischaemic and cold pain models) are discussed in some detail. Before doing so, the methods of quantifying the response to a painful stimulus are discussed.

Table 8.1. Some experimental pain stimuli.

Stimulus	References
Radiant heat to skin	10, 38, 58
Laser heat to skin	4, 5, 37
Cold immersion of limb	9, 21, 25, 27, 28, 43, 60, 61, 66–68
Electrical shocks to fingers, ear lobe, tooth pulp	7, 17, 22, 49, 56–58
Electrical shocks to nerve fibres	62
Hyper/hypotonic saline injected into muscle	65
Chemicals on catharidin blister base	2, 15
Pressure to bony prominences	26, 30
Pressure to skin folds	14
Ischaemic limb	20, 35, 36, 39, 40, 45, 50–52, 59, 70

Pain Rating

Many workers have attempted to get away from the vagaries of subjective assessments of pain and to provide more objective 'hard data'. However, skin conductance, autonomic variables, plasma catecholamines, cortisol and enkephalins have all failed to serve as satisfactory correlates of pain sensation. The measurement of evoked potentials in peripheral nerves and the brain, and electroencephalography have contributed enormously to our understanding of the neurophysiology of pain, and a number of studies have shown correlations between subjective reports and amplitude of certain potentials which are thought not to reflect merely the stimulus intensity.[4,5,7,22] Some studies in which subjective ratings have been combined with recording of evoked potentials have demonstrated effects of analgesics on both[11], but discrepancies between suppression of wave forms and subjective reports after administration of an analgesic have also been observed.[46] Both objective and subjective methods of pain measurement have been the subject of reviews[6,18], but suffice it to say that, to date, no satisfactory substitute has been found for the purely subjective report of pain which, despite all its drawbacks, seems to be the only means by which we can be sure that we are measuring pain intensity.

The verbal rating scale described by Keele[29] is simple and has, with minor modifications, been used extensively and very effectively by patients participating in clinical trials. Verbal descriptors have also been employed successfully, particularly in clinical trials.[54] However, the translation of words into numerical data which can be subjected to statistical analysis is problematic. The scales are fairly insensitive and are confounded by inter-individual differences in the value of words and readiness to recategorise. Furthermore, it cannot be assumed that the scale is linear, and statistical analysis of data is usually restricted to non-parametric methods. Visual analogue scales (VAS) are somewhat more difficult to comprehend, but trained volunteers do not usually have much difficulty, providing they are given very explicit instruction in how to use them. The use of different types of VAS[24,55] and the graphic representation of pain[48] have been extensively studied in patients. The choice of text and its position with respect to the line is critical to avoid skewed distributions, and the use of a scale along the length of the line is favoured by some workers. Logarithmic transformation of data from the VAS may be required, but generally the data can be subjected to analysis of variance.

The Submaximal Effort Tourniquet Test (SETT)

Some of the characteristics of ischaemic limb pain were described by Lewis, Pickering and Rothschild in 1931.[33] Beecher and co-workers[50,51,52], who made major contributions to our knowledge in this area thirty years ago, favoured the ischaemic stimulus because its duration resembles more closely that of 'pathological pain' than some other stimuli. After ex-sanguination of an arm and occlusion of the arterial blood supply with a tourniquet, isometric hand-grip exercise is performed. Rather than requiring the subjects to exercise until exhaustion or limited by pain, submaximal exercise is used to ensure that precisely the same amount of work is performed every time the subject is tested. The importance of standardising the exercise is underlined by investigations into the determinants of ischaemic muscle pain.[34] After cessation of exercise, ischaemic pain develops in the limb and gradually increases in severity until it becomes intolerable.

Analgesic effects of opioids[39,51] and transcutaneous electrical nerve stimulation[70] have been demonstrated by this technique, but early claims of demonstrations of analgesia with aspirin[50] have not been confirmed and many have found results too variable to be useful. The importance of standardisation of the technique was stressed by Sternbach.[59] A potential confounding factor for this model, and probably for all pain models, is the level of anxiety[19], which emphasises the importance of training volunteers to ensure that virtually all anxiety has been removed.

In an attempt to obtain greater sensitivity and reliability of SETT, we modified the technique with careful standardisation of exercise and experimental conditions. We have favoured the use of a visual analogue pain scale in the laboratory, but, rather than ask our volunteers to rate pain at fixed intervals, we have devised a computer-generated VAS so that trained subjects can rate pain intensity continuously for the duration of a pain test by moving a cursor along the VAS displayed on a monitor.

Volunteers perform the test seated in an air-conditioned, sound-proofed cubicle, observed from outside by means of closed-circuit television and in verbal communication with the operator by intercom. They are not permitted to wear a watch or to see a clock from the cubicle, the aim being that they lose track of time. First, the dominant arm is ex-sanguinated using an inflatable sleeve, and a tourniquet on the upper arm above the sleeve is then inflated. After removal of the sleeve, the subject performs intermittent isometric hand-grip exercises for 1 min on a dynamometer in time with an auditory signal. The maximum load is pre-set to 50% of his or her maximum grip-strength using a micrometer screw gauge. When this force is exerted, an electrical contact is made which lights an indicator bulb. On stopping exercise, the volunteer proceeds to rate pain intensity on the VAS, gradually moving the cursor from the 'No pain' to the 'Max pain' end of the scale as the pain increases. On reaching the 'Max pain' end, by which the subject indicates unbearable pain, the test is terminated and the tourniquet is released. The test generally lasts 5–10 min and can be performed at hourly intervals during the course of a study day, taking care to adhere to the same schedule on each occasion in order to avoid diurnal changes in pain sensitivity. Analgesia is assessed in terms of 'tourniquet time' and 'cumulative analgesia scores', the score being defined as the cursor distance from the 'Max pain' end of the line (*Figure 8.1*). Considerably more information than mere

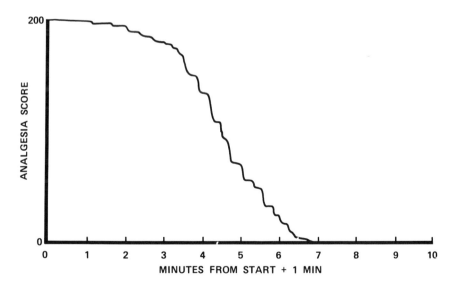

Figure 8.1. Graphic display of analgesia score of one subject performing SETT. Analgesia score: cursor position at no pain = 200 and maximum pain = 0. Tourniquet time: time from start of rating +1 min exercise.

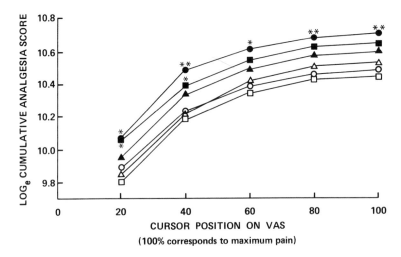

Figure 8.2. Mean overall analgesia scores for four sessions of SETT performed at hourly intervals following codeine 60 mg, ●; codeine 30 mg, ■; diazepam 5 mg, ▲; indomethacin 50 mg, □; indomethacin 25 mg, ○; and placebo, △ (n = 12); * and ** $p < 0.05$ and $p < 0.01$ with respect to placebo.

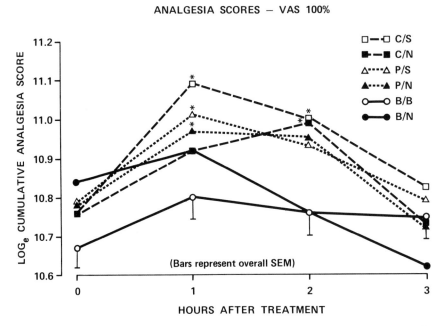

Figure 8.3. Mean cumulative analgesia scores of SETT performed at hourly intervals following oral administration of codeine 60 mg (C), matching placebo (P) or no treatment (B) with a concurrent intravenous infusion of saline (S), naloxone (N) or no infusion (B) (n = 12); * $p < 0.05$ with respect to B/B.

thresholds and tolerance can be obtained, as the cursor position is computed each second for the duration of the test. We analyse data from points 20, 40, 60, 80 and 100% along the VAS.

In a series of double-blind, placebo-controlled, randomised crossover studies, using 6–12 trained volunteers in each[39,40], we showed that the opioid dipipanone, in doses of 5 and 10 mg, and codeine 60 mg (*Figure 8.2*) have reliable statistically significant analgesic effects with the SETT model. Interestingly, as little as 30 mg codeine produced significant effects at low pain intensities (20–40% on the VAS), but no greater effect was seen at higher intensities, consistent with the clinical observation that low doses of analgesics can give adequate relief of mild pain. The opioid antagonist naloxone antagonised opioid-induced analgesia, but did not produce hyperalgesia (*Figure 8.3*).[40] In contrast to the finding of Grevert *et al.*[20], we did not demonstrate any antagonism of placebo analgesia, suggesting that endogenous opioids are not involved in ischaemic-limb pain or placebo analgesia under these conditions.

The coefficient of variation for this technique, using pre-drug sessions in three studies involving a total of 30 volunteers, was in the range 13–16% depending on which value was taken. The model seems to be quite specific for opioids, because the sedative effect of diazepam was not interpreted as analgesia and the non-steroidal anti-inflammatory drugs (NSAIDs) aspirin and indomethacin (*Figure 8.2*)[39], as well as paracetamol, did not exhibit any analgesic effects in this model. In fact, indomethacin, which did produce drowsiness, appeared to cause some hyperalgesia.

The Cold Pain (CP) Test

Immersion of a limb in ice-cold water has long been known to induce pain.[64] At 1–2°C, the initial sensation is of cold, but this is rapidly displaced by a burning sensation, which in turn changes into a deep aching pain which becomes progressively more intense. Unlike ischaemic pain, it does not continue to increase with the passage of time, but rather reaches a maximum within 60–90 sec and then remains constant at a level inversely related to temperature. If immersion continues, the limb usually becomes numb and the pain subsides, this process being known as adaption. It has been suggested that there are specific cold receptors and nociceptors situated in the walls of veins.[16]

The test is performed under similar conditions to those of the SETT. As with the ischaemic limb model, care is taken to train the subjects so that the element of anxiety is removed and pain rating is reasonably consistent before commencement of a study. The volunteer first immerses his or her dominant hand in a stirred water bath at 37°C for 2 min, before he or she transfers it to a stirred water bath at 2°C and immediately proceeds to rate the pain intensity on the VAS. Most volunteers consider the maximum pain to be severe but tolerable, so that the duration of the test can be fixed for all participants in a study, providing care is taken in preliminary training sessions to exclude a minority of volunteers who either cannot tolerate the pain or conversely feel no sensation of pain. Analysis of the results of a test of fixed duration (2 or 3 min) is somewhat simpler than for the variable length SETT, as a pain score rather than an analgesia score can be computed directly. Using the computerised VAS, effects of analgesics can be expressed in terms of absolute and cumulative 'pain scores', as well as 'times' taken to reach various points on the VAS.

The analgesic effect of opioids was shown using this model many years ago.[66] With the modifications described, we have demonstrated the sensitivity of this model to very small doses of opioids[43], with a coefficient of variation on baseline pain scores at 90 sec immersion being of the order of 10%. In a double-blind study in 12 subjects who performed the CP test before, and 1.5 and 3 h after being administered 2, 4 or 8 mg dipipanone or placebo, the

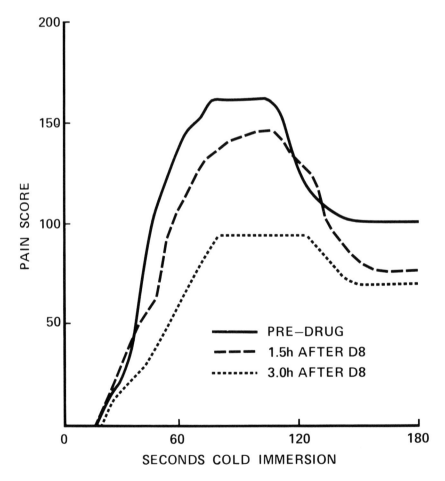

Figure 8.4. Pain ratings of one subject in three CP tests on an occasion when he received 8 mg dipipanone (D8).

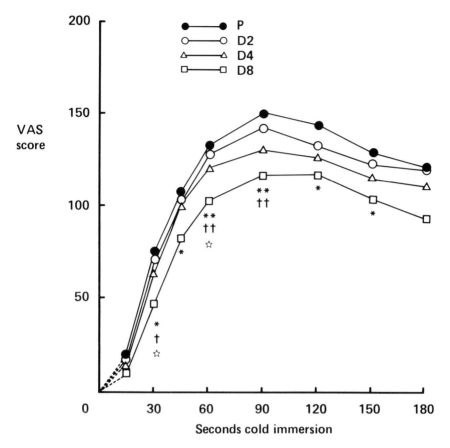

Figure 8.5. Mean pain scores during cold immersion 3.0 h after placebo (P), 2 mg, 4 mg or 8 mg dipipanone (D2, D4, D8, respectively) (n = 12); * $p<0.05$ and ** $p<0.01$ with respect to placebo, † and †† $p<0.05$ and $p<0.01$ with respect to D2, ☆ $p<0.05$ and ☆☆ $p<0.01$ with respect to D4.

highest dose reduced pain scores significantly compared with all other treatments; the 4 mg dose also reduced pain scores significantly compared with placebo and a dose–response relationship was evident (*Figures 8.4, 8.5* and *8.6*). Baseline arterial pressure was not affected by the opioid, but the pressor response to the CP test was significantly reduced (*Figure 8.7*), suggesting that the arterial pressure changes were secondary to pain rather than cold *per se*. Transcutaneous electrical nerve stimulation at various frequencies elevates cold pain threshold[27], possibly because endogenous opioids are involved. Hypnosis and acupuncture have also been used with effect in some subjects.[27,31] Like SETT, the CP model seems completely insensitive to the effects of NSAIDs.[28,60] Possible confounding factors affecting results with CP include the phase of menstrual cycle[21] and psychological traits and state.[9,23]

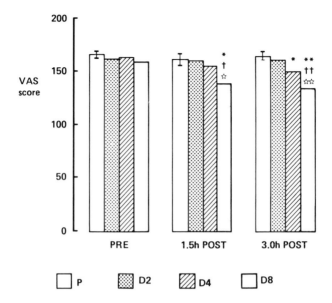

Figure 8.6. Mean maximum pain scores on CP test before, and 1.5 h and 3.0 h after placebo (P), 2 mg, 4 mg or 8 mg dipipanone (D2, D4, D8) (n = 12; bars represent overall standard error of mean); * and ** $p<0.05$ and $p<0.01$ with respect to placebo, † and †† $p<0.05$ and $p<0.01$ with respect to D2, ☆ and ☆☆ $p<0.05$ and $p<0.01$ with respect to D4.

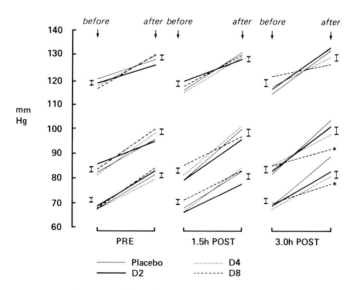

Figure 8.7. Mean systolic, diastolic and mean arterial blood pressures immediately before and after CP tests, before, and 1.5 h and 3.0 h after placebo, 2 mg, 4 mg or 8 mg dipipanone (n = 12, bars represent overall standard error of mean); * $p<0.05$ with respect to placebo.

Evaluation of an Enkephalin Analogue

443C81 (Tyr-D.Arg-Gly-Phe[4NO$_2$]-Pro-NH$_2$) is a synthetic enkephalin which penetrates the blood brain barrier poorly and exhibits antinociceptive activity in animals using models believed to reflect a peripheral site of action.[13] In a series of studies in healthy volunteers[41,42], using intravenous infusions at rates calculated to achieve pre-determined plasma concentrations and subsequently to maintain those values, we have demonstrated dose-related analgesia with this peptide (*Figure 8.8a,b*). There seemed to be a

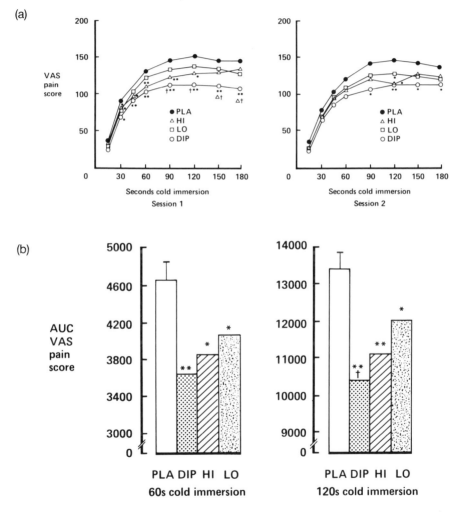

Figure 8.8. (a) Mean pain scores on 2 CP tests and (b) mean area under curve of pain scores at 60 and 120 sec cold immersion during first CP test performed at steady state concentrations of high- or low-dose 443C81, or at corresponding times after placebo or dipipanone (n = 12, bar represents overall standard error of mean); * and ** $p<0.05$ and $p<0.01$ with respect to PLA and † $p<0.05$ with respect to LO.

(a)

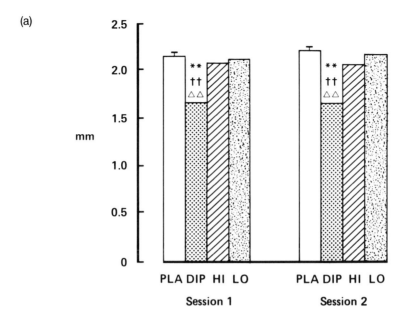

(b)

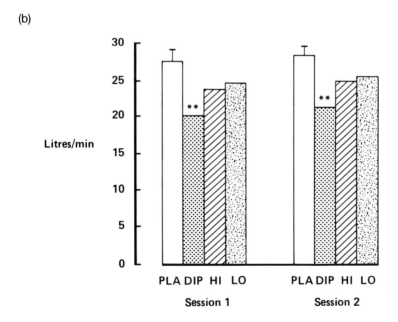

Figure 8.9. Central effects: mean values of (a) pupil diameters and (b) minute ventilation (at 60 mmHg $p\mathrm{CO_2}$) at steady state concentrations of high- or low-dose 443C81, or at corresponding times after placebo or dipipanone (n = 12, bar represents overall standard error of mean); **, † and △ $p<0.01$ with respect to PLA, LO and HI, respectively.

ceiling effect and the maximum analgesia was not as great as that of a standard therapeutic dose of the classic opioid dipipanone. Tests of central activity, which included measurement of pupil size (*Figure 8.9a*), respiratory response to rebreathing of carbon dioxide (*Figure 8.9b*), measurement of reaction time and subjective rating of sedation and mood, showed that, in contrast to dipipanone, the enkephalin was virtually devoid of central opioid effects, confirming the findings in animals. Vasodilator properties of 443C81 were demonstrated also, and the possibility was considered that the analgesic effects resulted from vasodilatation in the cold limb, but a study using the calcium antagonist nifedipine failed to show any non-specific analgesia. The enkephalin failed to elicit analgesia in the ischaemic limb model, which is consistent with a peripheral site of action as the painful limb is deprived of circulation and is therefore not exposed to the drug.

Models for Assessment of NSAIDs

The pain models discussed so far have proved totally insensitive to the action of NSAIDs. This is probably not simply a question of potency, as we have shown activity of quite small doses of codeine, but not even a trend toward pain relief after substantial doses of aspirin or indomethacin. Furthermore, our conception of relative potencies of analgesic drugs is often false as this depends very much on the stimulus. Thus, aspirin is an extremely poor analgesic for some visceral sources of pain, but is usually more effective than the most potent opioids against severe bone pain, particularly that associated with cancer. The explanation does not seem to lie in the fact that anti-inflammatory drugs may act at peripheral sites, because the CP model was sensitive to the peripherally-acting enkephalin. In addition, NSAIDs such as aspirin, zomepirac, ketoprofen and indomethacin have central effects.[8,12,47,63] It is more likely that the absence of effect is related to their mechanism of action which involves cyclo-oxygenase inhibition. Arachidonic acid metabolism is probably not involved in the pain stimuli studied to date.

The question remains whether there is any satisfactory model for demonstrating analgesia of aspirin-like drugs administered in normal therapeutic doses to healthy volunteers. There have been some claims of activity, particularly with models employing electrical stimulation as the stimulus. Using chains of square wave impulses of progressively increasing amplitude to stimulate the ear lobe with two silver balls, Stacher and his colleagues[56] found little effect from 550 mg of naproxen alone, but a potentiation of the elevation of pain threshold and tolerance produced by codeine 60 mg. Similar results were obtained on the pain threshold to a radiant heat stimulus applied to the volar aspect of the forearm. This group also demonstrated a dose-related increase of threshold and tolerance to the electrical stimulus, and of threshold to the thermal stimulus with diclofenac.[57] These studies have been conducted and analysed carefully, and the number of subjects has been comparatively large (48 in the latter study) while the magnitude of effect was small. Others have not been able to reproduce the results. Another study[49], reporting apparent analgesic effects of aspirin on pain scores obtained after electrical stimulation of the forefinger, can be criticised on statistical grounds.

Conclusions

If one avoids confounding factors, studies of experimental pain in trained, healthy volunteers can provide an extremely convenient and sensitive means by which to evaluate new putative opioid analgesics. Despite some positive results with non-steroidal anti-inflammatory drugs, a sensitive model for their analgesic properties has not yet been established.

References

[1] Beecher, H.K. Limiting factors in experimental pain. *J. Chronic Dis.*, **14**, 11–21, 1956.
[2] Bleehen, T. and Keele, C.A. Observations of the algogenic actions of adenosine compounds of the human blister base preparation. *Pain*, **3**, 367–77, 1977.
[3] Campbell, J.A. and Lahuerta, J. Physical methods used in pain measurements: a review. *J. Royal Soc. Med.*, **76**, 409–14, 1983.
[4] Carmon, A., Dotan, Y., and Sarne, Y. Correlation of subjective pain experience with cerebral evoked responses to noxious thermal stimulations. *Exp. Brain Res.*, **33**, 445–53, 1978.
[5] Carmon, A., Friedman, Y., Coger, R., and Kenton B. Single trial analysis of evoked potentials to noxious thermal stimulation in man. *Pain*, **8**, 21–32, 1980.
[6] Chapman, C.R., Casey, K.L., Dubner, R., Foley, K.M., Gracely, R.H., and Reading, A.E. Pain measurement: an overview. *Pain*, **22**, 1–31, 1985.
[7] Chatrian, G.E., Canfield, R.C., Knauss, T.A., and Lettich, E. Cerebral responses to electrical tooth pulp stimulation in man. An objective correlate to acute experimental pain. *Neurology*, **25**, 745–57, 1975.
[8] Chen, A.C.N. and Chapman, C.R. Aspirin analgesia evaluated by event-related potentials in man: possible central action in brain. *Exp. Brain Res.*, **39**, 359–64, 1980.
[9] Chen, A.C.N., Dworkin, S.F., Haug, J., and Gehrig, J. Human pain responsivity in a tonic pain model: psychological determinants. *Pain*, **37**, 143–60, 1989.
[10] Chery-Croze, S. Painful sensation induced by a thermal cutaneous stimulus. *Pain*, **17**, 109–37, 1983.
[11] Chudler, E.G. and Donk, W.K. The assessment of pain by cerebral evoked potentials. *Pain*, **16**, 221–44, 1983.
[12] Fink, M. and Irwin, P. Central nervous system effects of aspirin. *Clin. Pharmacol. Ther.*, **32**, 362–5, 1982.
[13] Follenfant, R.L., Hardy, G.W., Lowe, L.A., Schneider, C., and Smith, T.W. Antinociceptive effects of the novel opioid peptide 443C81 compared with classical opiates; peripheral versus central actions. *Br. J. Pharmacol.*, **93**, 85–92, 1988.

[14] Forster, C., Anton, F., Reeh, P.W., Weber, E., and Handwerker, H.O. Measurement of the analgesic effects of aspirin with a new experimental algesimetric procedure. *Pain*, **32**, 215–22, 1988.

[15] Foster, R.W. and Weston, K.M. Chemical irritant algesia assessed using the human blister base. *Pain*, **25**, 269–78, 1986.

[16] Fruhstorfer, H. and Lindblom, U. Vascular participation in deep cold pain. *Pain*, **17**, 235–41, 1983.

[17] Gabka, J. and Price, R.K.J. Tooth pulp stimulation: a method of determining the analgesic efficacy of meptazinol in man. *Br. J. Clin. Pharmac.*, **14**, 104–6, 1982.

[18] Gracely, R.H. Psychophysical assessment of human pain. *Adv. Pain Res. & Ther.*, **3**, 805–24, 1979.

[19] Graffenried, B. von, Adler, R., Abt, K., Nuesch, E., and Spiegel, R. The influence of anxiety and pain sensitivity on experimental pain in man. *Pain*, **4**, 253–63, 1978.

[20] Grevert, P., Albert, L.H., and Goldstein, A. Partial antagonism of placebo analgesia by naloxone. *Pain*, **16**, 129–43, 1983.

[21] Hapidou, E.G. and Catanzaro, D. de. Sensitivity to cold pressor pain in dysmenorrheic and non-dysmenorrheic women as a function of menstrual cycle phase. *Pain*, **34**, 277–83, 1988.

[22] Harkins, S.W. and Chapman, C.R. Cerebral evoked potentials to noxious dental stimulation: relationship to subjective pain report. *Psychophysiology*, **15**, 248–52, 1978.

[23] Hilgard, E.R. The alleviation of pain by hypnosis. *Pain*, **1**, 213–31, 1975.

[24] Huskisson, E.C. Measurement of pain. *Lancet*, 1127–31, 1974.

[25] Jalon, P.D.G. de, Harrison, F.J.J., Johnson, K.I., Kozma, C., and Schnelle, K. A modified cold stimulation technique for the evaluation of analgesic activity in human volunteers. *Pain*, **22**, 183–9, 1985.

[26] Jensen, K., Andersen, H.O., Olesen, J., and Lindblom, U. Pressure-pain threshold in human temporal region. Evaluation of a new pressure algometer. *Pain*, **25**, 313–23, 1986.

[27] Johnson, M.I., Ashton, C.H., Bousfield, D.R., and Thompson, J.W. Analgesic effects of different frequencies of transcutaneous electrical nerve stimulation on cold-induced pain in normal subjects. *Pain*, **39**, 231–6, 1989.

[28] Jones, S.F., McQuay, H.J., Moore, R. A., and Hand, C.W. Morphine and ibuprofen compared using the cold pressor test. *Pain*, **34**, 117–22, 1988.

[29] Keele, K.D. The pain chart. *Lancet*, 6–8, 1948.

[30] Keele, K.D. Pain-sensitivity tests. The pressure algometer. *Lancet*, 636–9, 1954.

[31] Knox, V.J. and Shum, K. Reduction of cold-pressor pain with acupuncture analgesia in high- and low-hypnotic subjects. *J. Abnormal Psychology*, **86**, 639–43, 1977.

[32] Lasagna, L. Analgesic methodology: a brief history and commentary. *J. Clin. Pharmacol.*, **20**, 373–6, 1980.

[33] Lewis, T., Pickering, G.W., and Rothschild, P. Observations upon muscular pain in intermittent claudication. *Heart*, **15**, 359–83, 1931.

[34] Mills, K.R., Newham, D.J., and Edwards, R.H.T. Fares, contraction frequency and energy metabolism as determinants of ischaemic muscle pain. *Pain*, **14**, 149–54, 1982.

[35] Moore, J.D., Weissman, L., Thomas, G., and Whitman, E.N. Response of

experimental ischemic pain to analgesics in prisoner volunteers. *J. Clin. Pharmacol.*, **11**, 433–9, 1971.

[36] Moore, P.A., Duncan, G.H., Scott, D.S., Gregg, J.M., and Ghia, J.N. The submaximal effort tourniquet test: its use in evaluating experimental and chronic pain. *Pain*, **6**, 375–82, 1979.

[37] Mor, J. and Carmon, A. Laser emitted radiant heat for pain research. *Pain*, **1**, 233–7, 1975.

[38] Nakahama, H. and Yamamoto, M. An improved radiant heat algometer and its application to pain threshold measurements in man. *Pain*, **6**, 141–8, 1979.

[39] Posner, J. A modified submaximal effort tourniquet test for evaluation of analgesics in healthy volunteers. *Pain*, **19**, 143–51, 1984.

[40] Posner, J. and Burke, C.A. The effects of naloxone on opiate and placebo analgesia in healthy volunteers. *Psychopharmacology*, **87**, 468–72, 1985.

[41] Posner, J., Dean, K., Jeal, S., Moody, S.G., Peck, A.W., Rutter, G., and Telekes, A. A preliminary study of the pharmacodynamics and pharmacokinetics of a novel enkephalin analogue [Tyr-D.Arg-Gly-Phe(4NO$_2$).-Pro.NH$_2$] (BW443C) in healthy volunteers. *Eur. J. Clin. Pharmacol.*, **34**, 67–71, 1988.

[42] Posner, J., Moody, S.G., Peck, A.W., Rutter, D., and Telekes, A. Analgesic, central, cardiovascular and endocrine effects of the enkephalin analogue [Tyr-D.Arg-Gly-Phe(4NO$_2$)-Pro-NH$_2$] (443C81) in healthy volunteers. *Eur. J. Clin. Pharmacol.*, **38**, 213–18, 1990.

[43] Posner, J., Telekes, A., Crowley, D., Phillipson R., and Peck, A.W. Effects of an opiate on cold-induced pain and the CNS in healthy volunteers. *Pain*, **23**, 73–82, 1985.

[44] Procacci, P., Zoppi, M., and Maresca, M. Experimental pain in man. *Pain*, **6**, 123–40, 1979.

[45] Roche, P.A., Gijsbers, K., Belch, J.J.F., and Forbes, C.D. Modification of induced ischaemic pain by transcutaneous electrical nerve stimulation. *Pain*, **20**, 45–52, 1984.

[46] Rohdewald, P., Derendorf, H., Drehsen, G., Elger, C.E., and Knoll, O. Changes in cortical evoked potentials as correlates of the efficacy of weak analgesics. *Pain*, **12**, 329–41, 1982.

[47] Schady, W. and Torebjork, H.E. Central effects of zomepirac on pain evoked by intraneural stimulation in man. *J. Clin. Pharmacol.* **24**, 429–35, 1984.

[48] Scott, J. and Huskisson, E.C. Graphic representation of pain. *Pain*, **2**, 175–84, 1976.

[49] Seki, T. Evaluation of effect of acetylsalicylic acid using electrical stimulation on the forefinger of healthy volunteers. *Br. J. Clin. Pharmacol.*, **6**, 521–4, 1978.

[50] Smith, G.M. and Beecher, H.K. Experimental production of pain in man: sensitivity of a new method to 600 mg of aspirin. *Clin. Pharmacol. & Ther.*, **10**, 213–16, 1968.

[51] Smith, G.M., Egbert, L.D., Markowitz, R.A., Mosteller, F., and Beecher, H.K. An experimental pain method sensitive to morphine in man: the submaximum effort tourniquet technique. *J. Pharmacol. Exp. Ther.*, **154**, 324–2, 1966.

[52] Smith, G.M., Lowenstein, E., Hubbard, J.H., and Beecher, H.K. Experi-

mental pain produced by the submaximum effort tourniquet technique: further evidence of validity. *J. Pharmacol. Exp. Ther.*, **163**, 468–74, 1968.

[53] Smith, R. The dynamics of pain. In *Problems of Dynamic Neurology*, L. Halpern (ed), 1–20, 1963.

[54] Sriwatanakul, K., Kelvie, W., and Lasagna, L. The quantification of pain: an analysis of words used to describe pain and analgesia in clinical trials. *Clin. Pharmacol. Ther.*, **32**,143–8, 1982.

[55] Sriwatanakul, K., Kelvie, W., Lasagna, L., Calimlim, J.F., Weis, O.F., and Mehta, G. Studies with different types of visual analogue scales for measurement of pain. *Clin. Pharmacol. Ther.*, **34**, 234–9, 1983.

[56] Stacher, G., Bauer, P., Schneider, C., Winklehner, S., and Schmierer, G. Effects of a combination of oral naproxen sodium and codeine on experimentally induced pain. *Eur. J. Clin. Pharmacol.*, **21**, 485–90, 1982.

[57] Stacher, G., Steinringer, H., Schneider, S., Mittelbach, G., Winklehner, S., and Gaupmann, G. Experimental pain induced by electrical and thermal stimulation of the skin in healthy man: sensitivity to 75 and 150 mg diclofenac sodium in comparison with 60 mg codeine and placebo. *Br. J. Clin. Pharmacol.*, **21**, 35–43, 1986.

[58] Stacher, G., Steinringer H., Winklehner, S., Mittelbach, G., and Schneider, C. Effects of graded oral doses of meptazinol and pentazocine in comparison with placebo on experimentally induced pain in healthy humans. *Br. J. Clin. Pharmacol.*, **16**, 149–56, 1983.

[59] Sternbach, R.A. The tourniquet pain test. In *Pain, Measurement and Assessment*, R. Melzack (ed), Raven Press, pp 27–31, 1983.

[60] Telekes, A., Holland, R.L., and Peck, A.W. Indomethacin: effects on cold-induced pain and the nervous system in healthy volunteers. *Pain*, **30**, 321–8, 1987.

[61] Telekes, A., Holland, R.L., Withington, D.A., and Peck, A.W. Effects of triprolidine and dipipanone in the cold-induced pain test, and the central nervous system of healthy volunteers. *Br. J. Clin. Pharmacol.*, **24**, 43–50, 1987.

[62] Torebjork, H.E., Ochoa, J.L., and Schady, W. Referred pain from intraneural stimulation of muscle fascicles in the median nerve. *Pain*, **18**, 145–56, 1984.

[63] Willer, J.C., Broucker, T. de, Bussel, B., Roby-Brami, A., and Harrewyn, J.M. Central analgesic effect of ketoprofen in humans: electrophysiological evidence for a supraspinal mechanism in a double-blind and crossover study. *Pain*, **38**, 1–7, 1989.

[64] Wolf, S. and Hardy, J.D. Studies on pain, observations on pain due to local cooling and on factors involved in the 'cold pressor' effect. *J. Clin. Invest.*, **20**, 521–33, 1941.

[65] Wolff, B.B. and Jarvik, M.E. Relationship between superficial and deep somatic thresholds of pain with a note on handedness. *Am. J. Physchol.*, **77**, 589–99, 1964.

[66] Wolff, B.B., Kantor, T.G., Jarvik, M.E., and Laska, E. Response of experimental pain to analgesic drugs. I. Morphine, aspirin and placebo. *Clin. Pharmacol. & Ther.*, **7**, 224–38, 1965.

[67] Wolff, B.B., Kantor, T.G., Jarvik, M.E., and Laska, E. Response of experimental pain to analgesic drugs. II. Codeine and placebo. *Clin. Pharmacol. & Ther.*, **7**, 323–31, 1965.

[68] Wolff, B.B., Kantor, T.G., Jarvik, M.E., and Laska, E. Response of experimental pain to analgesic drugs. III. Codeine, aspirin, secobarbital and placebo. *Clin. Pharmacol. and Ther.*, **10**, 217–28, 1968.

[69] Wolff, H.G., Hardy, J.D., and Goodell, H. Measurement of the effect on the pain threshold of acetylsalicylic acid, acetanilid, acetophenetidin, aminopyrine, ethyl alcohol, frichlovethylene, a barbiturate, quinine, ergotamine tartrate and caffeine: an analysis of their relation to the pain experience. *J. Clin. Invest.*, **20**, 63–7, 1941.

[70] Woolf, C.J. Transcutaneous electrical nerve stimulation and the reaction to experimental pain in human subjects. *Pain*, **7**, 115–27, 1979.

9. Analgesic Clinical Trials

W.S. Nimmo

The correct assessment of analgesic drugs depends on an ability to measure pain in a variety of clinical situations. Methods of measurement may overlap with those used in pain models (Chapter 8), but the pain stimulus is pathological. There is no precise definition of pain in these studies and there are many types of pain varying with different patient populations, diseases and settings. Pain is a complex and multi-dimensional perception involving sensory, affective and cognitive aspects.

Measurement of Pain

Pain measurement may be classified conveniently into two categories[4,16]: objective or observational, and subjective or self-report methods.

Objective or Observational

The observer clinician assigns numbers to scale a patient on one or more features of the pain. This may allow him to test the effect of a drug, to describe populations of patients or to characterise diseases or situations that cause pain. The scores allow comparison between patients or within the same patient under different circumstances (e.g. before and after an analgesic). Theoretically, this type of assessment can be carried out in animals. The criteria for scoring are well defined and independent of the patient.

This type of measurement has included observation of physiological variables and behaviour patterns (*Table 9.1*).

Problems exist with all of these objective methods of assessing pain. Physiological indicators, such as heart rate or arterial pressure, may correlate with nociception and the degree of tissue damage as well as occurring simultaneously with the pain, but they do not necessarily correlate exactly with the pain itself. There are many variables which influence the observations independently of the influence on the pain. Only when all other variables are controlled will these observations give additional information about the severity of the pain and any attempts to relieve it.

The measurement of plasma cortisol or catecholamines also lacks specificity as a measure of pain.[14] During trauma, there is a relationship with stress rather than pain. Noradrenaline concentrations have been used to measure

Table 9.1. Examples of objective methods used for the measurement of pain.

Physiological
Changes in heart rate, arterial pressure, cardiac output
Changes in respiration (e.g. forced expiratory volume in one
    second, forced vital capacity, peak expiratory flow)
Changes in blood cortisol or catecholamines

Neuropharmacological
Changes in beta endorphins
Changes in skin temperature

Neurological
Nerve conduction velocity
Evoked potentials

Behaviour patterns
Sighing, groaning, grunting
Demanding analgesics using a patient-controlled analgesia device

pain in patients with rheumatoid arthritis, but the extent of individual variation meant that the method could be used only in crossover trials where the patient acted as his own control.[9] Individual differences between treated and untreated patients were so small that it was necessary to collect urine for three days. However, in the acute pain of the post-operative period, there was no correlation between plasma catecholamine concentrations and linear analogue scores.[6]

It is assumed that beta-endorphin and beta-lipotropin are released during acute pain. Beta-endorphin is an endogenous opioid and some reports have identified an inverse relationship between beta-endorphin concentrations and acute pain severity.[17] However, beta-endorphin is released in response to stress as well as pain and its presence does not provide unequivocal evidence of the existence of pain.

Skin temperature has been used in the evaluation of some chronic pain states, partly because dysautonomias, including reflex sympathetic dystrophy, produce temperature changes of the skin of the affected limb. Also, arthritis may produce warmth in the overlying skin. However, there is not a close relationship between the temperature and the gradation of pain.

Short latency evoked brain potentials have been used to study peripheral neuropathology and for monitoring during surgery.[2] Long latency evoked potentials have been studied in volunteer studies and experimental pain, but not in patients or on clinical research.

A scanning technique, such as positron emission tomography, may allow the study of regional cerebral blood flow and glucose metabolic rate. At present, it must be used in conjunction with subjective reports of pain to produce results which have any meaning in the assessment of pain.

Subjective or Self-Report Methods

All of these measurements involve the patient making the assessment and assigning the numbers. They include single dimension and multi-dimension methods (*Table 9.2*).

Category scales are also known as simple descriptive scales (SDS) or verbal rating scales (VRS). There is little demand placed upon the patient and, in the simplest form, the patient is asked if he has pain or not. In other forms, it is necessary to choose the best word to describe the pain, e.g. mild, moderate or severe. This type of approach has been correlated with other methods (e.g. numerical scales) by some workers and it may have the least variation between subjects.[3] However, it lacks sensitivity. An alternative scale with more categories uses eight facial expressions to quantify pain.[7] The expressions range from happiness to extreme pain. These have correlated with visual analogue scales and may be useful in patients with language or mental difficulties.

The obvious advantages of the category scale are its simplicity and suitability for all patients. Its major disadvantages are its limited range and lack of sensitivity. Patients tend to use the middle of the range and this may limit the usefulness of the scale further. Statistical analysis should be appropriate for category scales and not continuous data.

Numerical rating scales involve asking the patient to rate his pain on a numerical scale. This provides a compromise in sensitivity between the simple descriptive scales and visual analogue scales. The range may be small or large (0 to 10, or 0 to 100). The categories are ranked easily and patients seem to understand the scales easily.

The intensity of the pain may be related to some other variable such as the intensity of a light, the loudness of a tone or the length of a line. This is known as cross-modality matching and its advantage is that equal intervals between levels are not assumed.[8]

A visual analogue scale (VAS) is a very commonly used method of pain assessment. Typically, a VAS consists of a 10 cm line with the patient scoring his pain by marking a point on the line. The ends of the line record two extremes such as 'no pain at all' and the 'worst pain imaginable'. The patient must be able to understand the two end points and must be free to indicate a point anywhere on the line. The line itself may be vertical or horizontal. It may also have graded descriptions of pain along the length of the line (being known as a graphic rating scale), although this is thought to limit choice and thus the sensitivity of the system.

The advantages of the VAS method are that the line represents a continuum of pain and the method is sensitive, reproducible and valid.

Table 9.2. Examples of subjective methods used in the assessment of pain.

Single-dimension methods
Category scales
Numerical rating scales
Visual analogue scales

Multi-dimension methods
McGill pain questionnaire
Dartmouth pain questionnaire
Pain inventory
Behavioural observational techniques
Pain diaries
Sickness impact profile

Disadvantages include difficulty of use by elderly patients, resulting in 11% of patients being unable to use the method.

Measurements from the visual analogue scale are made by a ruler, and the method is particularly suitable for measuring the effect of analgesic drugs as the pain intensity difference (PID) before and after treatment can be calculated and compared for two different analgesics. The sum of the pain intensity differences (SPID) may be shown to correlate with the dose of the analgesic drug.

The visual analogue scale has been modified to use electrical signals instead of a paper and pencil. The fundamental principle is unchanged, but the calculations may be automated and the results interpreted more frequently and more quickly.

Single observation tests are simple and efficient with few problems for the patients. The same test can be used repeatedly, and most patients and doctors understand what is being measured and how it can be interpreted. The numbers are produced directly and no elaborate scoring is required. Criticisms include their simplicity, as they may oversimplify the complex human experience of pain. They are influenced by other variables (e.g. emotions, tiredness or arousal) which are not measured separately. However, these scales remain the most used and accepted of all pain measurement techniques employed in analgesic clinical trials. There is no consensus view on which of the three tests is best. Each investigator should consider carefully which test suits him, his patients and the situation most appropriately.

In order to measure pain more comprehensively, a multi-dimensional approach is usually required. Each dimension or observation is an attribute of pain and each is measured using a visual analogue scale or a numerical rating scale. The response to one scale may affect that to another and therefore each response should be recorded without reference to the others.

The McGill pain questionnaire (MPQ) is the best known and most frequently used multi-dimensional scale.[12,13] This method tests pain in three main categories: sensory, affective and evaluative. Patients are given 20 sets of words that describe pain and are asked to select those sets that best describe the pain. There are 2–6 words in each set. The first ten sets indicate sensory quality, the next five the affective quality, the sixteenth is evaluative and the remaining four are miscellaneous. Methods exist to score each dimension and also to obtain a total score.

The Dartmouth pain questionnaire has been developed to supplement the MPQ by adding more information, including general feeling of pain, duration and intensity as well as behaviour influenced by the pain.

The MPQ seems to be reliable and valid as well as comprehensive. However, it takes 5–15 min to complete and some patients are unable to understand the vocabulary. The results must be interpreted as a whole and not in parts. Responses may be influenced by other persons present during the test, and on the whole the burden on the patient is greater than that of single observation tests. Nevertheless, the MPQ remains a test of first choice for measurement of the quality and character of a patient's pain.

A pain inventory may be used to obtain a shorter and more efficient measure of worst, average and current pain.[5] This method scales analgesic effect as well as the extent to which pain interferes with the quality of life.

Behavioural observation[11] depends on identifying any behaviour associated with pain and scoring it according to frequency, speed, rate or accuracy. This has been studied most often for patients with back pain and the behaviour includes rubbing the affected area, guarding movements and sighing. The scaling can be done with the help of video cameras.

Pain diaries are sometimes used by chronic pain clinics for behavioural self-reports. This is often activity-related and may involve recording a numerical rating scale for the pain and for any relief from medication for different activities, such as walking, sitting, reclining, etc. If completed daily, these diaries may be very good measures of pain during normal activities over a prolonged period of time, without the need for sophisticated equipment. A limitation is that the reliability is unknown and it may vary from patient to patient. Also, patients may record drug consumption up to 60% lower than actual usage.

The sickness impact profile (SIP)[1] is not specific for pain, but gives a general indication of health status. Three aspects are included – physical, psychosocial and overall – and chronic pain may be assessed by this method.

Sources of Error in Pain Measurement

Whatever the method of pain assessment, there are three main sources of error:

- Investigator bias. Any previous knowledge of the patient, illness or therapy may influence assessment. Therefore investigators must conduct all observations 'blinded' to the therapy and there should be placebo control as well as active comparator.
- Patient bias. This problem is greatest in subjective measurements. It is best minimised by precise instructions and guidance, standard conditions (e.g. no relatives present), and blinded treatment with placebo and active comparator comparisons. Bias is greatest when a patient is asked to remember pain over a period of time and this varies with the severity and nature of the current pain.
- Data collection and scoring. The placebo effect is great in analgesic clinical trials and the patient often reports a favourable outcome to please the doctor and to satisfy his expectations. The prospect of litigation, e.g. after trauma, may influence pain measurement.

Poor methodology or analysis of data should be avoided. There has been a tendency to analyse a category scale as if it were numerical and continuous. This should be avoided. Appropriate tests are necessary.[15]

Guidelines for Clinical Trials

Population

Clinical trials of analgesics can be carried out only if patients understand the instructions. Subjects should be of a suitable age (children and the elderly are much more difficult to study) and appropriate educational ability. A pilot

study of the proposed method of assessment may be required to ensure that it
is possible in the proposed population.

Goal of Measurement

Multiple observation methods are useful to characterise a particular pain and
to assess trends over a period of time, but they are not very useful to measure
acute pain or the effects of analgesics on acute pain. An appropriate
assessment must be determined in the light of the aim of the study and the
particular clinical situation.

Assess Different Options

The investigator should satisfy himself that the test he will use produces
reproducible results in his clinic and that there is good agreement between
patients. The range of measurements, and therefore intensity of pain, should
be wide, otherwise the scaling may not be meaningful. The method should be
sufficiently sensitive to detect differences between patients with known
differences in pain intensity and the effects of therapy. Pain scores must
approximate to a normal distribution or else non-parametric tests must be
used.

Know the Limits of the Tests Used

Although pain measurements may not be as precise or specific as other
measurements in clinical trials, meaningful data can be obtained if there is
careful attention to detail and a resistance to overinterpreting the data. In
addition, appropriate statistical tests must be used.

An excellent example of a simple category scale yielding precise information is illustrated in a simple study by Keats and others in 1950.[10] During the
first 30 hours after a surgical operation, patients were given injections of
drugs to relieve pain. At intervals of 45 min and 90 min after each injection,
they were interviewed and asked whether or not the pain had disappeared. If
they said 'yes' on both occasions, this was considered positive. Anything less
than this was counted as no effect at all.

In order to test the method, a constant dose of an unknown preparation
was given to each patient and varying doses of morphine were also given to
each patient. This was repeated some 50 times with each dose of morphine
and the percentage of positive effects was calculated. The difference between
this percentage for the unknown and the corresponding percentage for each
dose of morphine was calculated and plotted against the dose of morphine. A
line was fitted to the plotted points and the point on this line corresponding to
zero corresponded to 10.8 mg of morphine (*Figure 9.1*). In fact, the unknown
dose was 10 mg of morphine, so the error of the estimate obtained in this way
was 8%. The experiment was very simple and produced meaningful results.
The potency and efficacy of the unknown dose were estimated accurately
under practical conditions when the drug was being used as it was intended to
be used.

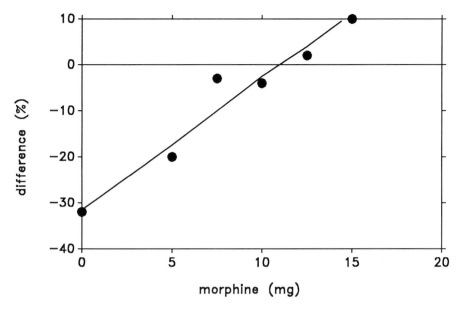

Figure 9.1. Comparison of analgesic potency of 'unknown drug' (actually 10 mg morphine) and of morphine. The x-axis is the dose of morphine, and the y-axis is the difference between per cent of responses to morphine and per cent of responses to the unknown. (Data redrawn after Keats *et al.*, 1950.[10])

Conclusion

Analgesic clinical trials rely for the most part on subjective observations. However, this is an indication for more careful preparation, collection and interpretation of data rather than despair. Meaningful results and conclusions are possible, although there have been few attempts to standardise methodology and to validate results.

References

[1] Bergner, M., Bobbitt, R.A., Carter, W.B., and Gilson, B.S. The sickness impact profile: development and final revision of health status measure. *Medical Care*, **19**, 787–805, 1981.
[2] Campbell, J.A. and Lipton, S. Intraspinal somatosensory evoked potential in man. In *Evoked Potentials: Neurophysiological and Clinical Aspects*, C. Morocutti and P.A. Rizzo (eds), pp 37–43, Elsevier, New York, 1985.
[3] Carlsson, A.M. Assessment of chronic pain. I. Aspects of the reliability and validity of the visual analogue scale. *Pain*, **16**, 87–101, 1983.
[4] Chapman, C.R. Assessment of pain. In *Anaesthesia*, W.S. Nimmo and G. Smith (eds), pp 1149–65, Blackwells, Oxford, 1989.
[5] Daut, R.L., Cleeland, C.S., and Flanery, R.C. Development of the

Wisconsin brief pain questionnaire to assess pain in cancer and other diseases. *Pain*, **17**, 197–210, 1983.

[6] Fell, D., Chmielewski, A., and Smith, G. Post-operative analgesia with controlled release morphine sulphate. *Br. Med. J.*, **285**, 92–4, 1982.

[7] Frank, A.J.M., Moll, J.M.H., and Hort, J.F. A comparison of three ways of measuring pain. *Rheumatology and Rehabilitation*, **21**, 211–17, 1982.

[8] Gracely, R.H., McGrath, P., and Dubner, R. Ratio scales of sensory and affective verbal pain descriptors. *Pain*, **5**, 5–18, 1978.

[9] Huskisson, E.C. Catecholamine excretion and pain. *Br. J. Pharmacol.*, **1**, 80–2, 1973.

[10] Keats, A.S., Beecher, H.K., and Mosteller, F.C. Measurement of pathological pain in distinction to experimental pain. *J. Appl. Physiol.*, **3**, 35–44, 1950.

[11] Keefe, F.J. and Block, A.R. Development of an observation method for assessing pain behaviour in chronic low back pain patients. *Behaviour Research and Therapeutics*, **13**, 363–75, 1982.

[12] Melzack, R. The McGill pain questionnaire: major properties and scoring methods. *Pain*, **1**, 277–99, 1975.

[13] Melzack, R. and Torgerson, W.S. On the language of pain. *Anaesthesiology*, **34**, 50–9, 1971.

[14] Moller, I.W., Rem, J., Brandt, M.R., and Kehlet, H. Effect of post-traumatic epidural analgesia on the cortisol and hyperglycaemic response to surgery. *Acta Anesthesia Scand.*, **26**, 56–8, 1982.

[15] Morton, A.P. and Dobson, A.J. Analysing ordered categorical data from two independent samples. *Br. Med. J.*, **301**, 971–3, 1990.

[16] Murrin, K.R. and Rosen, M. Pain measurement. In *Acute Pain*, G. Smith and B.G. Covino (eds), Butterworths, London, pp 104–32, 1985.

[17] Szyfelbin, S.K. and Osgood, P.F. The assessment of pain and plasma endorphin immunoactivity in burn children. *Pain*, **22**, 173–82, 1985.

10. Dose Taking *versus* Dose Timing in the Assessment of Drug Effects in Clinical Trials

J. Urquhart

Introduction

Peck[25] has recently analysed the reasons for variable drug response, noting that patient compliance vies with pharmacokinetics as the main source of such variance. Pharmacokinetic variability can be minimised by measuring drug concentration in plasma at a defined time after a defined dose on several occasions, thereby identifying those patients who are pharmacokinetic outliers and who, therefore, need adjustment of their dosage regimen. By the same token, poor compliance may be minimised by appropriate measurements, thereby identifying patients who need special attention or assistance to ensure correct dosing. Until recently, however, methods for measuring compliance have been unreliable and unable to provide a real-time record of dosing. New electronic methods for monitoring the time of dosage now form the basis of reliable estimation of compliance. In particular, they also make it possible to measure dose timing in outpatient clinical trials, turning variable compliance from a disadvantage into a new source of information about response to drugs. It is relevant in this context to consider the extent of poor and partial compliance in clinical trials, its clinical pharmacological correlates, and finally its implications for statistical analysis of trial results.

The Extent of Poor and Partial Compliance

The extent of poor and partial compliance in clinical trials has long been underestimated by the widespread use of 'pill counts'. With this method, the number of returned, unused unit doses is counted, subtracted from the number dispensed, divided by the number of days between dispensing and return, and the result is expressed as an average number of unit doses taken daily. Obviously, it cannot show when deviations occurred from the prescribed regimen, only the total number of missing unit doses and the presumed average daily dose.

Recently, Pullar *et al.*[30] compared pill counts with the results of a chemical marker method, and showed convincingly that the former 'grossly overestimate compliance'. This conclusion is confirmed by other data from Rudd *et al.*[32] and Cramer *et al.*[6] The main problem with the tablet count method is that the results are often grossly distorted by the discarding of dosage forms in a single act, just before the patient returns for a scheduled examination. This phenomenon has been termed the 'parking-lot effect' by investigators, who have found discarded tablets and capsules in parking lots outside their offices. It is one of several means by which patients disguise partial or poor compliance as good compliance.

Electronic monitoring methods[2,3,10,16,24,34] cannot prove actual ingestion of dosage forms, but they compile a timed and dated record of each use of the drug package as it occurs. It is a record that only a dedicated dissembler could falsify, because it requires sequential execution of the actions needed to remove a dose from the package, such as opening, closing, lid removal, tipping of the container or removal of a dosage form. A false record cannot be created retrospectively without totally reversing the engineering to subvert the electronic microcode by which the monitor operates. This would be a technically complex and costly task, far beyond the scope of either patients or physicians who might wish to create a false record of dosing times as they progress through a protocol.

Underdosing, the most common form of deviation from prescribed regimens, is revealed when the time for dosing passes without any electronic record of package use. For example, Kass et al.[14–17] have used an electronically monitored eyedrop dispenser that records time and date whenever there is concomitant cap removal and inversion of the dispenser. The coincidence of these two events does not prove that an eyedrop reached the eye, but, as the only way to place an eyedrop onto the eye is to invert the bottle with the cap removed, the failure of these two events to coincide at the appointed time is strong evidence that dosage did not occur.

Some solid dosage-form monitors record the time when individual unit doses are removed[3,10,22]; others record the time of package opening and closing.[2,34] For most applications, the simple recording of package opening and closing suffices to detect delays and omissions in dosing, which comprise the vast majority of deviations from the prescribed regimen.

The technique of monitoring one or more aspects of package use to indicate when dosing is occurring is called 'medication event monitoring'. While attention tends to focus on schemes for integrating microelectronics into various types of packages, an equally important component of medication event monitoring is the software system necessary to ensure the integrity of data as they are captured and stored in the monitors, and to transfer this information from the monitor into external data handling systems. The term 'system' in 'medication event monitoring system' denotes this vitally important aspect of measuring outpatient dosing.

'Taking' Compliance

Chemical marker and electronic monitoring methods both show a wide range of compliance among patients prescribed various kinds of chronic therapy. The overall average of prescribed doses taken is approximately 70%, with a range from 0% to approximately 120%. A more informative view shows that when patients are classified with respect to the fraction of prescribed doses taken during a month or more of observation, 50–60% take more than four-fifths, 30–40% take between two- and four-fifths, and the rest are more

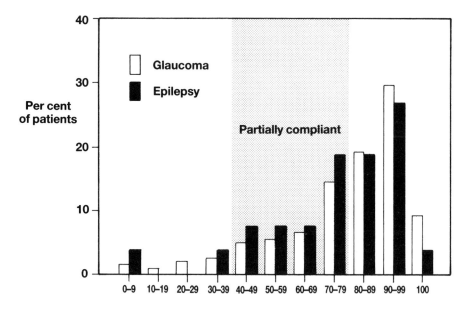

Compliance
(Per cent of prescribed doses taken)

Figure 10.1. Distributions of compliance (measured as dose-taking, without consideration of dose-timing) in 174 patients with glaucoma, taking pilocarpine eyedrops q.i.d. and monitored for four weeks,[14] and in 24 patients with epilepsy taking a variety of oral anti-epileptic drugs and monitored for five months.[6] (Copyright 1990, APREX Corporation; reproduced with permission.)

or less equally divided between those who take less than two-fifths of prescribed doses and those who take more doses than pre-scribed.[3,6,13–15,17–19,30]

One of the striking aspects of reliable compliance measurements is the similarity of the findings across different types of chronic drug therapy. For example, *Figure 10.1* shows the similar distribution of compliance (as a percentage of prescribed doses taken) in the treatment of glaucoma and epilepsy. *Figure 10.2* indicates the general situation regarding compliance.

'Timing' Compliance

The foregoing discussion referred to 'taking compliance', which does not consider the often important factor of dose timing. Many patients who take most or all of their prescribed doses do so at intervals that are substantially different from those directed. For example, Rudd *et al.*[31] found that only a small minority of patients took more than two-thirds of their doses within 9–15 h of one another, despite taking more than 80% of prescribed doses in a ten-week trial or two antihypertensive agents. Instead, most dosed themselves at intervals that alternated between 16–18 h and 6–8 h. If a drug

The Compliance Pie Revealed by
Electronic Monitoring Data

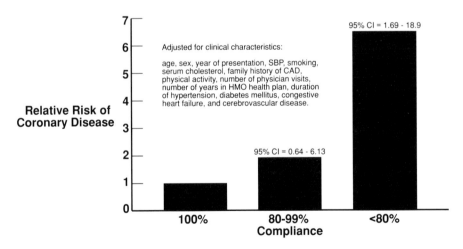

A. The majority take the drug almost as prescribed. Their dose timing is often different than assumed, which may undermine efficacy.

C. A small fraction takes practically no drug at all - with little or no drug response.

B. Partial compliers usually respond partially to the drug. Sometimes their dosing halts for several days, which may trigger adverse rebound effects.

D. Another small fraction takes more drug than prescribed - often with little or no extra efficacy, sometimes with extra side-effects.

Figure 10.2. Pie chart showing the approximate distributions of compliance (measured as dose-taking, without consideration of dose-timing) in major areas of chronic drug therapy. (Copyright 1990, APREX Corporation; reproduced with permission.)

product intended to be dosed twice-daily has a duration of action of only 12–13 h, drug action will cease during the latter part of the 16–18 h dosage intervals. Whether such recurring gaps in drug action have an adverse

Adjusted for clinical characteristics:

age, sex, year of presentation, SBP, smoking, serum cholesterol, family history of CAD, physical activity, number of physician visits, number of years in HMO health plan, duration of hypertension, diabetes mellitus, congestive heart failure, and cerebrovascular disease.

Relative Risk of Coronary Disease

95% CI = 1.69 - 18.9
95% CI = 0.64 - 6.13

100%   80-99%   <80%
Compliance

Figure 10.3. The relationship between compliance with prescribed systemic beta-blocker drugs and relative risk of incident coronary heart disease (defined as new onset angina, myocardial infarction (fatal and/or non-fatal), or sudden death) in patients with hypertension. Compliance was measured by comparing the actual time of prescription refill with the time predicted from the amount of drug previously dispensed and the directions for its use. CAD = coronary artery disease, SBP = systolic blood pressure. (Based on data in Table 5 of Psaty *et al.*[29]).

influence on the course of therapy depends on the clinical condition and the drug. Such interruptions in dosing may also cause rebound effects.

Clearly gaps in therapy will be much longer when patients omit doses, particularly when skipping several doses in sequence. In this event, not only do patients fail to receive the benefits of treatment, but the risk from rebound phenomena is much greater. A prominent example is the risk of myocardial infarction and other manifestations of coronary heart disease in patients who abruptly discontinue beta-blockers. Not surprisingly, the risk of incident coronary heart disease is increased 4–6 fold in patients who take less than 80% of prescribed beta-blockers for hypertension (*Figure 10.3*).[29]

How Scheduled Visits to the Doctor Distort Patterns of Compliance

An important factor that acts to increase compliance is knowledge of an impending scheduled visit to the physician.[6,7,14,17] This factor is variously referred to as the 'toothbrush effect', by analogy to the tendency to brush one's teeth just before visiting the dentist, or 'white coat compliance'.[11] The pre-visit surge in compliance creates a number of distortions in the clinical assessment of the patient, such that measurements made during the consultation may not reflect values obtained when compliance is at its usual level.[11]

An important casualty of the pre-visit surge in compliance is the attempt to use therapeutic drug monitoring – the measurement of plasma drug concentrations – as a measure of compliance. Unless the drug being monitored has an exceptionally long half-life, one or two days of correct dosing is sufficient to restore drug concentrations to the therapeutic range. Thus, as the time for a scheduled blood sampling draws near, compliance usually improves, and the measured drug concentration gives little or no indication of the usually prevailing dosing pattern. Cramer *et al.* have clearly demonstrated how this mechanism operates to preclude use of blood concentration measurements of anti-epileptic drugs as a measure of compliance.[6,7]

The scheduling of frequent consultations with the patient may be a useful stratagem to secure a period of good compliance, but it is expensive and is probably sooner or later offset by the Hawthorn effect. The pre-visit surge in compliance threatens the external validity of the results of clinical trials when their design includes substantially more frequent visits than are likely to prevail in clinical practice.

Clinical Pharmacological Correlates of Poor and Partial Compliance

Some Basic Features of Dose–Response Relations

As discussed by Edgar[8], most dose–response relationships are non-linear. They can usually be characterised by a minimum effective dose, a range of doses within which the relation of effect to dose is fairly steep, and then a more or less asymptotic approach to a maximum effect which cannot be exceeded by further large increases in dose. The curves relating different effects of the same drug to dose are not necessarily parallel, and each effect will be characterised by a different minimum effective dose. Thus, one can expect to find a low range of doses within which no discernible effects of the drug are elicited. At higher doses, only one or two of the drug's effects will be elicited, and at still higher doses, several effects will be elicited. At yet higher doses, most or all of a drug's recognised effects may be produced.

Interpretation of Variable Compliance as Variable Dosing

If the recommended dose of a drug is set correctly and rationally, and if the drug has a reasonable therapeutic index, a patient who is fully compliant with the prescribed regimen will experience nearly full therapeutic effect and little or no side effects. If, however, the patient is only partially compliant – taking only part of the prescribed doses during the treatment interval – drug responses at that time will be incomplete or only partially expressed. If the patient takes only a small fraction of prescribed doses, little or no drug effect may occur. Thus, if the clinician has measured compliance and knows of these variations in dosing, this can help to explain variations in drug response.

The prevalence of poor or partial compliance is so high that it should be the first consideration when inadequate drug responses or therapeutic failures are observed. When the clinician overlooks or has no data on variations in dosing, however, variations in drug response may be erroneously ascribed to 'biological variation', 'a non-responder patient', 'variable drug absorption', 'variable disposition', and the like.

The pre-visit surge in compliance may obscure the effects of chronic underdosing. It depends on whether a few days of more or less correct dosing suffice to restore measurable drug actions to full-dose levels. For example, a few days of correct dosing with most antihypertensive agents may restore elevated blood pressure to normal, but would not prevent or reverse cardiac, renal or vascular pathology arising from the usually elevated blood pressure.

Fixed-Dose Trials as Natural Experiments in Dose Ranging

One of the more important consequences of variable compliance for clinical trials is the conversion of fixed-dose trials into 'natural' dose-ranging studies.

A 'natural' experiment is one not purposefully designed, but comprising a set of spontaneously occurring circumstances that may, with certain caveats, be interpreted as an experiment. The concept and interpretation of natural experiments pertinent to human health and disease lie within the purview of epidemiology. Proper interpretation of natural experiments requires understanding of the reasons for the naturally occurring variation that have, in the first place, created the experiment.

Variable compliance means that patients self-select their own dosing levels. There are a number of reasons for variable compliance, the most common being simple negligence. The measurement of compliance with placebo in a placebo-controlled drug trial reveals the combined effects of two recognised factors that negatively influence compliance, namely negligence and a distaste for self-administering the dosage form, e.g. swallowing tablets or capsules.

When one finds identical distributions of compliance with both the active agent and the placebo among participants in randomised, blinded, placebo-controlled trials, this signifies that the effects of the drug have had no additional net impact, one way or the other, on compliance. For this reason, it is important to measure compliance with placebo as well as with the test agent. (It is also important that identical procedures be applied to both active and placebo groups to prevent inadvertent unblinding of the trial.) If there is some action of the drug that discourages compliance, it will tend to shift the distribution of compliance downward among recipients of the active agent in a placebo-controlled trial. Eugene Stead once commented that it is difficult for drug treatment to make an asymptomatic patient feel better. This aphorism is apt when assessing the impact of drug therapy for chronic, asymptomatic conditions, where the patient is asked to put up with a certain unpleasantness in exchange for the promise of some long-term benefit of a probabilistic or actuarial nature. On the other hand, if the drug has perceptible benefits, they may act to facilitate compliance among recipients of the active agent relative to recipients of placebo.

In the Helsinki Heart Study the distributions of compliance were essentially identical between recipients of active and placebo.[23] The prevalence of poor compliance due to negligence may be judged from the results of a special study of compliance done as part of that trial. Three methods were used to assess compliance in a large sample of the participants: (a) a count of returned, unused dosage forms; (b) urinary excretion of marker quantities of digoxin that had been added to the dosage forms; (c) in-depth interview of the patients. Considering the combined results of all three methods, the investigators concluded that only 57% of participants were satisfactorily compliant.[22]

The Lipid Research Clinics Coronary Primary Prevention Trial illustrates how unpleasant drug side-effects can result in more patients registering lower compliance levels in the active compared to the placebo limbs of the trial.[21] The active agent, cholestyramine, is given in large doses and has the harmless but prevalent side-effects of dyspepsia, bloating and flatulence. In a different clinical setting, Kruse *et al.*[18] have provided a striking example of the impact of side effects on compliance. Patients prescribed a seven-day course of ethinyl estradiol as part of a diagnostic test for infertility, showed a wide range of poor and partial compliance that demonstrated an inverse correlation between the severity of oestrogen-induced nausea and the extent of compliance.

In other instances, disease severity may influence compliance. This effect was observed by Coates *et al.*[4], who showed that patients with more severe heart failure complied better with a prescribed regimen of exercise than did patients with less severe failure. They attributed this difference to a greater expectation of benefit among those with more severe heart failure.

In short-term therapy, the patient's perception that cure has been achieved may lead to premature cessation of dosing. On the other hand, patients frustrated by the lack of promised benefit may discontinue treatment. To interpret these various results, one needs to measure the time history of patients' dosing, and to ask patients why they deviated from the prescribed regimen.

Every trial should include procedures for discovering the main reasons for poor and partial compliance with the agent(s) and regimen(s) being tested. A first step is to examine the distributions of compliance with the various agents and regimens. When the distributions of compliance are found to be similar for active and placebo, it is likely that negligence is the main source of variable compliance, although an aversion to swallowing solid dosage forms may contribute. Some of this information can be obtained by direct questioning of patients during or after the trial, and some by searching for systematic differences in patient characteristics at different levels of compliance, as described by Coates et al.[4]

Procedures for enquiring about compliance, or for trying to improve it in the course of a trial, must be applied equally to all participants, with careful regard to the risk of inadvertent unblinding.

Statistical Issues

Statistical concerns about using compliance data as an explanatory variable have their origin in the fact that compliance is self-selected by patients after randomisation, and may, therefore, introduce bias into the interpretation of the trial's results. While this is true, it is only one of several important considerations that must be balanced in the imperfect world of trial analysis. Another consideration is that the trial is a test of the drug's actions, and they depend directly, if the drug has any activity at all, on both dose-taking and dose-timing. A further consideration is that, as already indicated, patterns of poor, partial and good compliance are strikingly similar across many types of chronic drug therapy, suggesting a general negligence when the regimen requires repetitive self-administration without some kind of immediately perceptible benefit, reward or reinforcement. Many people are simply not very good at executing the repetitive task of dosing correctly.

One should, however, be vigilant in seeking additional reasons for variable compliance, not only to identify and understand bias, but for the practical clinical reasons of understanding why erroneous dosing is occurring and the extent to which it interferes with therapeutic action. Such information is basic to any attempt to take practical steps to improve therapeutic results by improving compliance.

Trialists' *Bête Noire* on Using Compliance Data in Trials Analysis

The most often cited example of compliance-linked bias in the interpretation of clinical trials relates to the Coronary Drug Project (CDP) trial of clofibrate.[5] In this five-year, randomised, placebo-controlled, multi-centre trial, a lipid-lowering agent of marginal efficacy was tested in patients with proven coronary heart disease.[1] A prior myocardial infarction was one of the inclusion criteria. At enrolment, about one-fifth of the patients had electrocardiographic signs of myocardial ischaemia and at least half were taking other cardiovascular drugs, including nitrates, diuretics, antihypertensives and inotropics.[1] As in any trial, the use of other potent drugs constitutes an important source of variation in morbidity and mortality. Thus, there will be:

- Variable response to correctly taken non-trial drugs.
- Variable compliance to such drugs.
- Variable prescribing of non-trial drugs, suggesting variable degrees of severity of the underlying disease at the time of enrolment.

Although randomisation is supposed to balance the average effect of all of these sources of variance, each added source of unallocated variance robs the trial of power.

Compliance was monitored with clofibrate and with placebo, but not with the non-trial drugs. Presumably, however, compliance with placebo reflected compliance with non-trial drugs.

The mortality during the ensuing five years of the trial was rather high, which is consistent with the existence of coronary heart disease and the history of prior myocardial infarction at the time of patient enrolment. Indeed, as reviewed previously[33], mortality was 7–9 times higher in the CDP trial than in subsequent trials of lipid-lowering agents which, by design, enrolled patients with abnormal lipid levels, but *without* clinical evidence of coronary heart disease.[12,21,23]

The analysis of the CDP trial showed a strong association between placebo compliance and mortality (*Table 10.1*). There was a 40% lower mortality in patients who took more than 80% of placebo doses than in patients who took less than 80% of placebo doses; the same large difference was seen in patients receiving clofibrate. Clearly, clofibrate had no detectable effect, but the huge difference in mortality associated with placebo compliance is striking – it constitutes the largest 'effect' on overall mortality seen in any of the trials of lipid-lowering agents.

The investigators argued from these results that it is unsound to use compliance data as an explanatory variable.[5] With the benefits of hindsight and information from later, better-designed trials of lipid-lowering agents, however, one might say that the CDP investigators would have done better to make four points about the role of compliance in their trial. First, the breakdown of the data by compliance shows that clofibrate is ineffective at each of two different levels of estimated dose, adding to the weight of evidence that the drug is ineffective. Second, they might have pointed out the weakness in the methods used to estimate compliance (see Appendix 1). Third, they might have considered the statistical problems of a study design that sought to measure weak effects (of lipid modification) against a background of serious disease known to result in high morbidity and mortality. Fourth, they might have focused attention on the imposing array of powerful non-trial drugs that the patients were taking, correctly in some instances, incorrectly in others.

Table 10.1. Five-year mortality in CDP patients by treatment group, according to five-year averages of estimated compliance.

Compliance (% of prescribed doses estimated to have been taken)	Treatment group			
	Clofibrate		Placebo	
	Patients (No.)	Mortality (%)	Patients (No.)	Mortality (%)
≥80	708	15.0	1813	15.1
<80	357	24.6	882	28.2
All patients	1065	18.2	2695	19.4

The third and fourth points relate to the most likely explanation for the apparent association between placebo compliance and mortality. Thus, placebo compliance reflects compliance with other agents that the patient is taking – in this instance, the diuretics, inotropics, antihypertensives, antiarrhythmics and other powerful non-trial medications that so many of the trial participants were taking for their coronary heart disease. Anyone who has cared for patients with advanced coronary heart disease and congestive heart failure knows that poor compliance with such medications is a source of poor outcome. It is surprising that this obvious factor was ignored in the interpretation of this trial.

Thus, the compliance data, flawed as they are, serve to reveal a major problem in the design of the Coronary Drug Project trial. Concomitant use of potent non-trial medications poses a statistical problem akin to that of a high tare in a weighing operation. Whether or not one chooses to use compliance data in various kinds of analyses, the finding of a strong association between placebo compliance and outcome is a warning signal that variable compliance with non-trial medications has occurred and has been a major source of variance. It is trouble enough to have a large placebo effect, but worse that a placebo effect on a major endpoint appears to be compliance-dependent.

Some authors[27] have sought to emphasise compliance behaviour as a major factor in health outcome. Before invoking such a vague and even mystical influence, one should first look carefully at the full range of tasks that patients are asked to perform in the trial, and evaluate the links between compliance with placebo and compliance with the regimens for performing those tasks. The tasks include the taking of concomitant non-trial medications, exercise, diet and the maintenance of personal hygiene. Each of these is a potential factor that influences the outcome, factors that patients ought to attend to, but may do so to varying degrees only. Each factor has a more or less understood mechanistic basis for influencing morbidity or mortality. After the effects of these factors have been evaluated, any residual association of placebo compliance with trial endpoints might be attributed to the non-specific influence of compliance behaviour.

What about Bias?

Increasing sophistication in trials design and interpretation has taught everyone to be wary of biases in assigning causality in any kind of test carried out on humans. Although one should be wary of bias, the identification of a bias is no reason to suspend further efforts to interpret the results of a trial. With respect to compliance, one should be even more wary of generalising from the results of trials in which the distribution of compliance behaviour is not representative of that in normal clinical practice. Much more needs to be learned about the differing incentives to comply in trials as opposed to in general practice. The matter of informed consent to placebo controls, for example, alerts the patient to the substantial chance of receiving an ineffective treatment, which is scarcely an incentive to comply when it is inconvenient to do so. One of the difficulties of applying results of intent-to-treat analyses to the practice situation is the implicit assumption of equal distributions of compliance in the two situations. This is an assumption which should not be made without data to support it.

   When compliance is distributed similarly between active and placebo, simple comparisons using compliance strata between active and placebo recipients can indicate several very practical aspects of drug effect:

1 The average effects of correctly following the recommended regimen.
2 The average effects in patients with the most common pattern of erroneous dosing.
3 The average effects in patients with the second most common pattern of erroneous dosing.
4 Exceptional effects in patients with exceptional patterns of dosing.
5 The overall average effects in all patients randomised to receive the drug, irrespective of compliance.

This approach was followed in the Lipid Research Clinics Coronary Primary Prevention Trial of cholestyramine[5] and is reflected in the US labelling of the agent.[26]

   Note that the overall average effects of the drug will depend on the extent to which drug actions are influenced by the most commonly occurring patterns of erroneous dosing and the proportions of patients in the first four groups listed above. An unusually negligent group of patients enrolled into a trial will, for example, result in relatively few patients in group 1 above, with more in groups 2–4, and a lower overall average value of drug effect. On the other hand, a group of exceptionally meticulous dosers enrolled into a trial will result in a higher all-patient average value of drug effect.

   Lasagna[20] has called attention to the impact that a charismatic investigator can have in encouraging patients to participate in clinical trials. One of the quantitative reflections of an investigator's charisma is that more of his or her patients comply well, in respect to both dose taking and dose timing. This factor, in turn, can give rise to between-centre differences in drug effect – another source of variation which good compliance data can help to explain.

Oral Contraceptive Evaluation: a Useful Precedent

Investigators in the oral contraceptive field were among the first to recognise the impact of variable compliance on the results of clinical trials by defining two types of effectiveness[28]:

- Method-effectiveness – indicated by the results in group 1.
- Use-effectiveness – indicated by the results in group 5.

This distinction was made because oral contraceptives were quickly recognised as having a virtually zero failure rate when taken correctly, and it was clearly important to distinguish between method failures and use failures. As time passed and the initially excessive oestrogen doses were steadily reduced, contraceptive efficacy became progressively more dependent on strict maintenance of the prescribed dosing schedule.

   Other fields of medicine have lacked this clarity of view in distinguishing the two types of treatment failure, such that therapeutic failures are common and too readily assigned to 'biological variability'.

Estimating the Risk of Bias in Using Compliance as an Explanatory Variable

If there is no evident association between placebo compliance and outcome or other measure of efficacy, and if the distributions of compliance are similar in placebo and active groups, there is unlikely to be any residual bias in the simple interpretation of variable compliance as variable dosing. However, if these conditions are not met, it may be useful to select patients, after the trial, from the various compliance strata and test their responses to the drug under strictly supervised dosing.

What to do when the Distributions of Compliance are Dissimilar between Active and Placebo Limbs

Side effects of drugs may discourage compliance, over and above the effects of simple negligence. In effect, patients 'vote with their mouths' about how much of the drug they take and when. Kruse et al.[18] have recently given a dramatic example of how drug-induced nausea can drastically reduce compliance. The question, however, is what to do when such effects occur?

The first and most important thing to do is to learn why the distributions are dissimilar: what was it about the drug that led patients to take fewer or lower doses, and what can be done about it? If, for example, it is mainly a problem of dosage form palatability, the problem may be minimised by reformulation. If it is a side-effect problem that is in some way linked to peak post-absorptive concentrations of drug, reformulation in a rate-controlled dosage form may help.

A second consideration is to learn whether the effect was large enough to have unblinded the trial.

A third consideration is to try to learn how the patients at the low end of the dosing spectrum differ from those at the higher end. They may, for example, be much more sensitive responders to the drug. This type of inquiry is one way to approach the study of population pharmacodynamics.

Efron and Feldman[9] have described a procedure for compensating for the effects of differential compliance, in a new type of primary analysis that identifies a portion of the drug dose–response relation from compliance–response data. It includes a statistical method for adjusting for different distributions of compliance between active and placebo.

Other examples of dose–response relations described from compliance-stratified data are to be found in the report of the Helsinki Heart Study[23] and in the US labelling of cholestyramine[26], based on the findings of the Lipid Research Clinics Coronary Primary Prevention Trial.[21]

A Practical Example of Variable Compliance in a Cooperative Patient

An example may help to illustrate how negligence and 'voting with one's mouth' may interact. It illustrates several principles:

- Pharmacological understanding does not compete effectively for priority in a busy schedule.
- Various reasonable considerations can take precedence over prescribed regimens.
- Concomitant use of more than one agent complicates matters, not only because there is more to forget, but also because the dictates of one regimen sometimes collide with those of another.

Here is the example.

This author takes cholestyramine and an HMG-CoA synthetase inhibitor to control a life-long predisposition to high cholesterol levels resistant to dietary control. This treatment is made desirable by the need to minimise the risk of development of atheromata in coronary bypass grafts. As a physician, I self-prescribe and periodically self-monitor the results of the treatment. Both professional and personal health interests have given me a good deal of information on the cholesterol-lowering drugs, and my doctor–patient relationship is, of course, good. However, with a busy life I am sometimes negligent in following the regimen I know to be ideal. I endeavour to take one or two 4 g doses of cholestyramine at a time, aiming for a total of 24 g, reasonably widely spaced throughout a 24 h period. However, dosing at bedtime or later usually awakens me with dyspepsia, so my policy is not to take the drug after about 21.00. Thus, I have to take my 3–6 doses during the time that separates my awakening and 21.00. There is, however, need to space morning and evening doses of the HMG-CoA synthetase inhibitor, either 1 h before or 2 h after cholestyramine, because of possible interference with absorption. I maintain a policy that the doses of the synthetase inhibitor take precedence over those of cholestyramine, and consider that it is pointless to take more than 8 g of cholestyramine at a time. I also maintain an interval of at least 4 h between cholestyramine dosing. When I delay doses of cholestyramine, I simply run out of time to take the necessary doses before 21.00. Thus, a combination of factors interact to produce a day-by-day dosing record that is often at marked variance with the evenly spaced total daily dose of 24 g of cholestyramine that I would ideally like to take.

As Kass noted in patients taking concomitant q.i.d. pilocarpine and b.i.d. timolol, compliance with the b.i.d. regimen in the two-drug regimen is considerably improved relative to monotherapy with the b.i.d. drug.[15] My experience is consistent: the effort to take the cholestyramine serves to maintain an awareness of 'need to dose', thereby benefiting my compliance with the b.i.d. synthetase inhibitor.

Conclusion

Much new information on out-patient compliance with drug treatment has been gleaned in the four years since data began to be published on the results of real-time, electronic monitoring. Most of this information has become available in the past year, following the introduction in late 1988 of the first commercially-available electronic monitors of dosing with tablets and capsules for oral use.

There is still much to be learned, but it is now clear that wide variations in compliance, due mainly to extensive negligence, are often the single greatest source of variance in drug response. With due attention to possible biases, the association between variable compliance and variable drug responses can be interpreted as dose–response information, thereby enriching the interpretation of clinical trials, particularly in respect to questions of optimal regimen design.

Reliable, real-time measurements of compliance can not only account for an appreciable proportion of the variance in drug response, but can also be used to improve the understanding of how drug effects – both beneficial and undesirable – depend on both dose quantity and dose timing.

APPENDIX 1: Problems with Compliance Measurement in the Coronary Drug Project Trial of Clofibrate

The procedures followed for ascertaining compliance allowed observers to estimate rather than count the number of returned dosage forms, complicating this unreliable method with observer bias. Furthermore, patients receiving drug, but not placebo, could be identified as being poorly compliant from routine assays for a clofibrate metabolite in urine samples. On the basis of results of this assay, centres were notified about poorly compliant patients, and asked to urge the patients to do better. A patient could only be so identified if he was a recipient of drug, not placebo, and, therefore, this procedure partly unblinded the study, and probably increased the likelihood of observer bias in the estimation of returned dosage form count.[1] For further discussion on these points, see Urquhart.[33]

References

[1] Anon. The coronary drug project: design, methods and baseline results. *Circulation*, **47** (Suppl. I), 11–179, 1973.
[2] Averbuch, M., Weintraub, M., and Pollock, D.J. Compliance monitoring in clinical trials: the MEMS device. *Clin. Pharmacol. Ther.*, **43**, 185, 1988.
[3] Cheung, R., Dickins, J., Nicholson, P.W., Thomas, A.S.C., Smith, H.H., Larson, H.E., Deshmukh, A.A., Dobbs, R.J., and Dobbs, S.M. Compliance with antituberculous therapy: a field trial of a pill-box with a concealed recording device. *Eur. J. Clin. Pharmacol.*, **35**, 401–7, 1988.
[4] Coates, A.J.S., Adamopoulos, S., Meyer, T.E., Conway, J., and Sleight, P. Effects of physical training in chronic heart failure. *Lancet*, **335**, 63–6, 1990.
[5] Coronary Drug Project Research Group. Influence of adherence to treatment and response of cholesterol on mortality in the coronary drug project. *N. Engl. J. Med.*, **303**, 1038–41, 1980.
[6] Cramer, J.A., Mattson, R.H., Prevey, M.L., Scheyer, R.D., and Ouellette,

V.L. How often is medication taken as prescribed? A novel assessment technique. *JAMA*, **261**, 3273–7, 1989.

[7] Cramer, J.A., Scheyer, R.D., and Mattson, R.H. Compliance declines between clinic visits. *Arch. Int. Med.*, **150**, 1509–10, 1990.

[8] Edgar, B. See Chapter 5, this volume.

[9] Efron, B. and Feldman, D. Compliance as an explanatory variable in clinical trials. *J. Am. Stat. Assoc.*, **86**(413), 7–26, 1991.

[10] Eisen, S.A., Woodward, R.S., Miller, D., Spitznagel, E., and Windham, C.A. The effect of medication compliance on the control of hypertension. *J. Gen. Intern. Med.*, **2**, 298–305, 1987.

[11] Feinstein, A.R. Editorial. *Arch. Int. Med.*, **150**: 1377–8, 1990.

[12] Frick, M.H., Elo, O., Haapa, K., Heinonen, O.P., Heinsalmi, P., Helo, P., Huttunen, J.K., Kaitaniemi, P., Koskinen, P., Manninen, V., Maenpaa, H., Malkonen, M., Manttari, M., Norola, S., Pasternack, A., and Pikkarainen, J. Helsinki heart study: primary-prevention trial with gemfibrozil in middle-aged men with dyslipidemia. *N.Engl. J. Med.*, **317**, 1237–45, 1987.

[13] Jeiven, M.L. and Anderson, F.A. Electronic compliance monitoring in oral contraceptive clinical studies. *Program & Symposia Abstracts, 4th Annual Meeting of Amer. Assoc. Pharm. Scientists*, Atlanta, A66, 1989.

[14] Kass, M.A., Gordon, M., and Meltzer, D.W. Can ophthalmologists correctly identify patients defaulting from pilocarpine therapy? *Am. J. Ophthalmol.*, **101**, 524–30, 1986.

[15] Kass, M.A., Gordon, M., Morley, R.E., Meltzer, D.W., and Goldberg, J.J. Compliance with topical timolol treatment. *Am. J. Ophthalmol.*, **103**, 188–93, 1987.

[16] Kass, M.A., Meltzer, D., and Gordon, M. A miniature compliance monitor for ophthalmology. *Arch. Ophthalmol.*, **102**, 1550, 1984.

[17] Kass, M.A., Meltzer, D., Gordon, M., Cooper, D., and Goldberg, J. Compliance with topical pilocarpine treatment. *Am. J. Ophthalmol.*, **101**, 515–23, 1986.

[18] Kruse, W., Effert-Kruse, W., Rampmaier, J., Runnebaum, B., and Weber, E. Compliance with short-term high-dose oestradiol in young patients with primary infertility – new insights from the use of electronic devices. *Agents and Actions Suppl. 29. Risk Factor for Adverse Drug Reactions: Epidemiological Approaches*, 105–15, 1990.

[19] Kruse, W. and Weber, E. Dynamics of drug regimen compliance – its assessment by microprocessor-based monitoring. *Eur. J. Clin. Pharmacol.*, **38**, 561–5, 1990.

[20] Lasagna, L. In *First International Symposium on Compliance Monitoring*, Heidelberg, June 6, 1988 (13 papers). Summary available from APREX.

[21] Lipid Research Clinics Coronary Primary Prevention Trial results: (I) Reduction in incidence of coronary heart disease; (II) The relationship of reduction in incidence of coronary heart disease to cholesterol lowering. *JAMA*, **251**, 351–74, 1984.

[22] Maenpaa, H., Manninen, V., and Heinonen, O.P. Comparison of the digoxin marker with capsule counting and compliance questionnaire methods for measuring compliance to medication in a clinical trial. *Eur. Heart J.*, **8** (Suppl. I), 39–43, 1987.

[23] Manninen, V., Elo, M.O., Frick, H., Haapa, K., Heinonen, O.P., Heinsalmi, P., Helo, P., Huttunen, J.K., Kaitaniemi, P., Koskinen, P.,

Maenpaa, H., Malkonen, M., Manttari, M., Norola, S., Pasternack, A., Pikkarainen, J., Romo, M., Sjoblom, T., and Nikkila, E.A. Lipid alternations and decline in the incidence of coronary heart disease in the Helsinki Heart Study. *JAMA*, **260**, 641–51, 1988.

[24] Norell, S.E., Granstrom, P.A., and Wassen, R. A medication monitor and fluorescein technique designed to study medication behaviour. *Acta Ophthalmol*, **58**, 459, 1980.

[25] Harter, J.G. and Peck, C.C. Chronobiology: suggestions for integrating it into drug development. *Annal. N.Y. Acad. Sci.*, **618**, 563–571, 1990.

[26] Physicians' Desk Reference. *QUESTRAN (cholestyramine)*. Medical Economics Co., Oradell, NJ, pp 726–7, 1990.

[27] Pledger, G.W. Compliance in clinical trials: impact on design. In *Epilepsy Research* (Suppl. I), D. Schmidt and I.E. Leppik (eds), Elsevier, Amsterdam, pp 125–33, 1988.

[28] Potter, L.S. Oral contraceptive compliance and its role in the effectiveness of the method. In *Patient Compliance in Medical Practice and Clinical Trials*, J.A. Cramer and B. Spilker (eds), Raven Press, New York, pp 195–207, 1991.

[29] Psaty, B.M., Koepsell, T.D., Wagner, E.H., LoGerfo, J.P., and Inui, T.S. The relative risk of incident coronary heart disease associated with recently stopping use of beta-blockers. *JAMA*, **263**, 1653–7, 1990.

[30] Pullar, T., Kumar, S., Tindall, H., and Feely, M. Time to stop counting the tablets? *Clin. Pharmacol. Ther.*, **46**, 163–8, 1989.

[31] Rudd, P., Ahmed, S., Zachary, V., Boston, C., Bonduelled, B. Improved compliance measures: application in an ambulatory hypotensive day trial, *Clin. Pharmacol. Ther.*, **48**, 676–85, 1990.

[32] Rudd, P., Byyny, R.L., Zachary, V., LoVerde, M.E., Titus, C., Mitchell, W.D., and Marshall, G. The natural history of medication compliance in a drug trial: limitations of pill counts. *Clin. Pharmacol. Ther.*, **46**, 169–76, 1989.

[33] Urquhart, J. Patient compliance as an explanatory variable in four selected cardiovascular studies. In *Patient Compliance in Medical Practice and Clinical Trials*, J.A. Cramer and B. Spilker (eds), Raven Press, New York, pp 301–22, 1991.

[34] Urquhart, J. and Chevalley, C. Impact of unrecognised dosing errors on the cost and effectiveness of pharmaceuticals. *Drug Information J.*, **22**, 363–78, 1988.

11. Clinical Pathology Measurements: The Detection and Significance of what is Abnormal

P.J. Wyld

Introduction

In the assessment of new drugs, considerable resources are devoted to the performance of clinical trials. At all stages of assessment, phase I to phase IV, a part of this effort is concerned with the measurement of a variety of chemical and haematological values. Not only does new technology present new options for the choice of methodology of existing assays, but it also expands the range of analyses it is possible to measure. The expansion of the variety and number of tests results in increasing amounts of data which require analysis and interpretation. Critical reasoning in the selection of tests will help to make subsequent analysis of the results easier. This process should include a number of considerations, including the assessment of the clinical value, choice of methodology and discussion of the expected results in the knowledge of the methods of analysis. In the event, it may be necessary to reappraise analytical methods if unanticipated changes occur during the study.

It is the purpose of this review to consider the steps which should be taken in determining the significance of the laboratory test results, along with all other measures of safety or efficacy made during a study.

Reasons for Performing Laboratory Tests

Laboratory tests are carried out for many reasons. These have been considered by a number of authors[10] and an amalgamation of several ideas is shown in *Table 11.1*. In practice, laboratory tests should occur for either of two reasons: analysis of pharmacodynamic effects or as part of the screening for adverse events. These two indications may be predictable from pre-clinical testing and from knowledge of the type or class of drug. Unexpected reactions to drug administration may be detected by the net of investigations being cast widely. Sometimes regulatory authorities will require this approach during the early development of a drug. The efficiency of this type of screening may be limited, particularly in early clinical trials, by the small number of volunteers or patients studied.[6] This may present only a relatively small view of the potential treatable population.

Table 11.1. Reasons for performing a laboratory investigation.

1. To be complete
2. They say . . .
3. Will get into trouble if we do not
4. Academic
5. If it were my mother, father, son, etc.
6. We might as well while we are doing the other
7. Few dare argue . . . FDA

Range of Tests

There has been a steady expansion of the range of tests which may be performed. New technologies mean that it is frequently possible to make an analysis widely available, sometimes before wide experience makes it possible to determine the values which differentiate normality from abnormality.

There are many examples of these developments. During the past ten years, haematological analysers have made it possible to measure platelet parameters, such as platelet volume, routinely.[11] Hitherto, this was a measure used exclusively by researchers.[4,5] It has taken some years since the measure of platelet volume was introduced for its correct interpretation in a number of disease states to be made.[7]

Another example is new methodology for the calculation of MCHC by haematology analysers. Mean corpuscular haemoglobin concentration (MCHC) measures the concentration of haemoglobin in the erythrocytes. In the past, this was the most accurate index of red cells because it did not involve a red cell count. The red cell count was the least accurate parameter using existing technology, i.e. a counting chamber. MCHC is susceptible to variations in the haematocrit because of trapped plasma. Most commonly seen in iron deficiency is the now 'normal' electronic MCHC caused by an overestimated haematocrit. As a result of this, it is better to consider a measured index, like mean corpuscular volume (MCV) when considering iron deficiency. Generally a good correlation exists between MCV and disease states.[12] The clinical value of the MCHC has had to be reconsidered.

Clearly, the introduction of a new analyte in a study may create a problem not only in measurement for the laboratory, but also in interpretation for the clinician. Our own experience with analyses for which there is inadequate prior evaluation is that they frequently cloud the interpretation of data familiar to the investigator. That such a situation should arise at all may be difficult to comprehend. There is a great desire to gain information on a new product. It is perhaps excusable that companies and regulatory authorities should wish to collect data, the significance of which may only become apparent at a later date.

Understanding the Analysis

Not all those involved in clinical trials need have detailed knowledge of assay methods, but everyone who participates in the trial design must consider methodology and its limitations. *Table 11.2* shows a number of haematological disorders in which it is clear that correct interpretation of the data requires, not only automated cell counting, but also further examination of the red cell indices, which may include a blood film.

While every attempt is made to consider the result in advance of the measurement, it is not unusual to be left with questions about interpretation. This is most frequent when new analytes are being measured.

Table 11.2.

Disease	Findings on blood film
Compensated acquired haemolytic anaemia	Spherocytosis, polychromasia, erythrocyte agglutination
Hereditary spherocytosis	Spherocytosis, polychromasia
Haemoglobin C disease	Target cells
Thalassaemia trait	Hypochromia, target cells
Elliptocytosis	Elliptocytes
Lead poisoning	Basophilic stippling
Incipient pernicious anaemia or folic acid deficiency	Macrocytosis, with oval macrocytes, hypersegmented neutrophils
Multiple myeloma, macroglobulinaemia	Rouleaux formation
Malaria, babesiosis	Parasites in the erythrocytes
Consumptive coagulopathy	Schizocytes
Mechanical haemolysis	Schizocytes
Severe infection	Relative increase in neutrophils; increased band forms, left shift
Infectious mononucleosis	Atypical lymphocytes
Agranulocytosis	Decreased neutrophils, relative increase in lymphocytes
Allergic reactions	Eosinophilia
Chronic lymphocytic leukaemia (early)	Relative lymphocytosis
Acute leukaemia (early)	Blast forms

Biological and Analytical Variation

There are many pre-analytical causes of variation which may be introduced into a clinical trial. Prolonged venous stasis during venepuncture may affect blood calcium concentrations, and stress and exercise can introduce variation in a number of relatively common analyses. For example, plasma creatine phosphokinase concentrations may become raised by up to 30% above the upper limit of normal levels after moderate exercise.[8] A raised concentration may continue for several days.

Reference ranges taken from the published literature may be related to a specific population that frequently is not similar to the one immediately under consideration in the trial. Ideally, patients with a disease should be compared with a group of subjects who are in other ways similar, but specific-disease free. This will include both healthy and 'non-healthy' subjects.[9] It is thus legitimate to compare patients attending a hospital clinic with others attending the same hospital as outpatients. It is preferable to compare similar populations with each other. This allows for a more accurate assessment of the reference range and thus any determination of normality and abnormality.

Clearly, when we wish to see whether changes occur in relation to drug administration, we must make more than one analysis. During the trial of a new medicine, measurements are usually made before, during and after the dosing period. When a single blood sample from a patient is assayed several times, identical values are not found on each occasion. Results follow a normal distribution and the standard deviation or coefficient of variation is termed the 'analytical imprecision'. This may be calculated from internal and external quality assurance schemes in all participating laboratories. These schemes provide participants with an accurate assessment of their own method and allow comparison with the use of the same method by other laboratories. Such schemes are an essential part of laboratory procedure.

In the UK, the National External Quality Assurance Scheme (NEQAS) in haematology has a system for laboratory classification according to performance in the measure of a particular test. Using the distance from the median value, a deviation index (DI) is calculated using the formula:

$$DI = \frac{(M - \text{result})}{S}$$

where M is the median and S the estimated standard deviation.

A particular result may then be classified into four categories: excellent, good, satisfactory/borderline and check calibration/check instrumentation. Satisfactory and better performances in the laboratory should give additional confidence to the interpreting physician and the importance of this cannot be overestimated.

Variation also occurs within a subject from day to day. This may be cyclical or random. Patterns of change may emerge during monitoring which may appear to relate to the drug. Changes in the subject's condition must be considered if other causes can be excluded.

For all these reasons it may be of additional value to know the 'critical difference' for a particular parameter. Critical differences are calculated from the coefficients of variation of analytical and within subject variation according to the following formula:

$$\text{Critical difference} = K \{CV_a + CV_w\}$$

where K is a factor dependent on the probability level selected, CV_a is the coefficient of analytical variation and CV_w is the coefficient of within-subject variation.

The higher the critical difference for a measured parameter, the greater the change must be to indicate a 'true' or 'clinically significant' change. Thus, when considering small changes, it becomes more likely that the change is due to one or a combination of causes of clinically 'insignificant variability'. Some examples of average critical differences are sodium 3%, potassium 14%, amylase 30%, calcium 5%, haemoglobin 8%, white blood cell count (WBC) 32%, and platelets 25%. Critical differences appear to be more than a statistical curiosity.[13] It has been shown that physicians respond to larger changes than the critical difference would suggest is reasonable. This may be due to a lack of awareness of true differences or because the clinician requires to be more than 95% certain that a difference exists. Whatever the reason, it is an indicator that the physician should have this additional information made available to him in an easily digestible form. Clinicians, when uninfluenced by such information, have a higher threshold for abnormality or degree of change than is suggested as reasonable by statistical analysis of the data.

Costongs et al.[3] found that large analytical variances in a study of short- and long-term intra-individual variation resulted, at least in part, from the use of different analysers. This should be a caution to all those considering multi-centre studies, where any assessment of variability should take account of the performance of different laboratories.

Specificity and Sensitivity

No special consideration should be given to the so-called 'routine' haematology and clinical chemistry assays performed in the course of a study. It is just as important with 'routine' assays to determine the relevance of the result to the study being undertaken. It is equally necessary to measure the importance of a test by understanding its sensitivity, specificity and predictive value.

New, improved technology has increased the sensitivity of many tests carried out in clinical laboratories. The possible predictive value of any test depends not only on the sensitivity and specificity of the assay, but also on the prevalence of any abnormality in the population under study. In the conduct of clinical trials, tests are performed to detect adverse events. The prevalence of any abnormality may be as high as 1 in 40. The positive predictive value of a test will show variation dependent, not only on the specificity, but also on the prevalence. An example is shown in *Table 11.3*. Over 30% of the results in this example will give a false positive result when the prevalence is 1 in 40.[9]

Table 11.3.

Sensitivity (%)	Specificity (%)	Prevalence of Event (%)	Positive Predictive Value (%)
85	98	20	91
85	98	5	69

Selection and Frequency of Measurement

The selection of an assay in a study should be part of a careful process of consideration of the study drug and the relation of the assay to this. One of

Table 11.4. Abnormalities* of tests of liver function in normal volunteer residential studies.

	Placebo	*Active*
Ast	2/166 (1.2%)	17/265 (6.4%)
Alt	6/166 (2.6%)	26/265 (13.6%)
AP	1/166 (0.6%)	0/265 (0%)
Bi	0/166 (0%)	5/265 (1.8%)
GGT	3/149 (2.2%)	5/242 (2.0%)
Total	12/1223 (1%)	63/1302 (5%)

* An abnormal result was any result outside the normal range developing during the study.

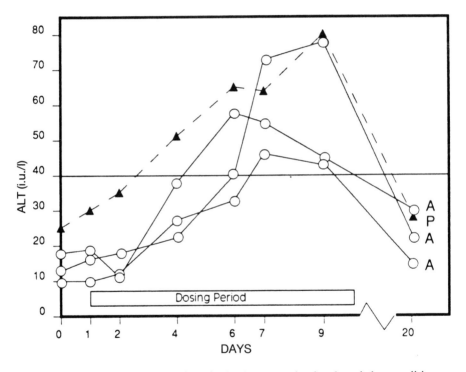

Figure 11.1. ALT concentrations (i.u./l) of volunteers who developed abnormalities during a study. A = active, P = placebo. Normal range is <40 i.u./l.

the most frequent examples of an abnormal result in any study is a test of liver function.

In early clinical trials, there are guidelines that recommend not only the tests to be performed, but also the frequency with which they should be performed.[1] Criteria for interpretation and classification of results are also available which may allow comparisons to be made between studies. We have recently reviewed our own experience of abnormalities of liver function tests in residential volunteer studies (*Table 11.4*).

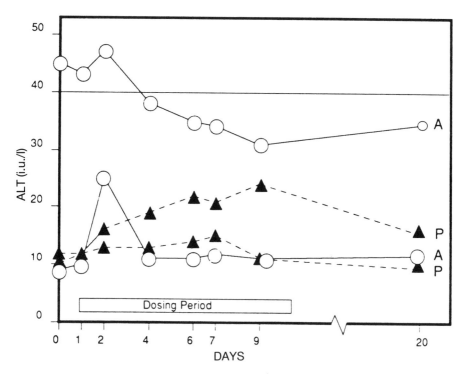

Figure 11.2. ALT concentrations (i.u./l) of volunteers whose concentrations were within the normal range during the study. A = active, P = placebo. Normal range is <40 i.u./l.

Our analysis shows a higher frequency of abnormalities of aspartate transaminase (Ast) and alanine transaminase (Alt) concentrations in the plasma of volunteers receiving active drug, compared with those receiving placebo, in five different studies during periods of 4–16 days under standard conditions of diet and restricted physical activity.

In *Table 11.4* the changes that occurred in those receiving placebo, as well as those receiving active drug, are shown. Abnormalities occurred more frequently in those receiving active drug.

An example of data from one of these studies reveals two patterns of changes in Alt concentrations during a study of ten days' dosing. These are indicated by *Figures 11.1* and *11.2*. *Figure 11.1* shows four volunteers whose Alt concentrations went outside the normal range at some time during the study. In *Figure 11.2* the concentrations of Alt in the four volunteers that did not exceed the upper limit of normal are shown. In each group of four, there was a mixture of active and placebo treatment.

There are a number of ways one may interpret these results:

- There are more subjects with abnormalities in the active (3/5) than in the placebo (1/3) groups.
- Mean values at different time points show no statistically significant differences between active and placebo by repeated measure Anova.

- Changes do not all follow the same pattern. Those of one subject appear to show improvement before the end of dosing.
- Changes occur in one subject in the placebo group.
- The magnitude of the changes in the placebo group is similar to that seen in the active group. This may mean that a factor other than the test drug was responsible for the change.

Overall there are difficulties with the interpretation of these data, and a combination of clinical interpretation and statistical analysis is necessary. Small numbers and wide inter-subject variation make such a process far from simple.

Interpretation of Results

Clinical researchers may judge laboratory results in a variety of ways. Broadly considered, there are clinical assessments and statistical assessments, which may include specific reference to:

- Results outside the reference range.
- Changes in results.
- More than one allied abnormality of a result, e.g. among tests of liver function (transaminases Ast and Alt).
- Changes beyond a predetermined value, e.g. 10% above upper limit of reference range.
- Changes the investigator believes are drug related. This may include interpretation of transient changes or trends in changes of values.

The clinical interpretation of a value is frequently the final arbiter in the determination of significance of the result. In early clinical trials, the assistance that the statistician may provide is often limited by the number of determinations performed.

In large-scale studies, a number of different methods for analysis have been used. Ciccolunghi et al.[2] and have shown the value of clinical interpretation in a method for analysis of laboratory investigations, described for large-scale multi-centre clinical trials. Their scheme for classification of abnormalities (*Table 11.5*) is similar to that proposed and used by others. All classifications have the potential for forcing the selection of an inappropriate category simply because of the restrictions any classification places on the interpreter. Overall, the methods proposed are time-consuming in both the pre-trial and analytical stages, but they represent clearly the principles upon which any proper analysis of results should be based.

Conclusion

Determination of the normality of laboratory data relies largely on clinical interpretation in all stages of clinical trials. From the outset of any trial, understanding the test is of major importance in the future determination of

Table 11.5. Classification of laboratory abnormalities.

Category	Criteria used for assignment
1.1 Spontaneous variation	1. Abnormality present for a maximum of 1–2 visits which was either temporary despite continued treatment or occurred on the last visit only and was minimal. A progressively increasing abnormality over 3–4 visits was never considered to be spontaneous variation 2. No relevant unwanted effects, other laboratory abnormalities or concomitant disease 3. No relevant concomitant medication 4. No comment or action by investigator
1.2 Laboratory or recording error	1. Usually a single aberrant value or, if more than one, evidence of centre effect 2. No relevant unwanted effects, other laboratory abnormalities or concomitant disease 3. No relevant concomitant medication 4. No comment or action by investigator
2. Minimal change of no probable clinical significance	1. Abnormality represents such slight deviation from the norm that it is obviously of no clinical significance 2. No relevant unwanted effects, other laboratory abnormalities or concomitant disease 3. No relevant concomitant medication 4. No comment or action by investigator
3. Relevant concomitant disease or operation	1. Relevant concomitant disease (recorded by investigator and/or evidenced by pre-treatment abnormality in another laboratory test) or operation present at time of abnormality 2. Any unwanted effects or laboratory abnormalities present must confirm this impression 3. No relevant concomitant medication 4. Confirmatory comment or action by investigator

(cont.)

Table 11.5 (*cont.*) Classification of laboratory abnormalities.

Category	Criteria used for assignment

4. Possible drug effect:
  4.1 No relevant concomitant medication taken
  4.2 Relevant concomitant medication taken
	1. Abnormality progressively increased during trial
	2. Relevant unwanted effects and other laboratory abnormalities present
	3. Confirmatory comment or action by investigator. Treatment should not be prematurely discontinued for laboratory abnormality unless relevant concomitant disease or operation present
	4. Abnormality, other than minimal, present at the last visit only

5. Probable drug effect	1. Abnormality progressively increases during trial 2. Relevant unwanted effects and other laboratory abnormalities present 3. No relevant concomitant medication taken or disease present 4. Confirmatory comment or action by investigator. Treatment may be prematurely discontinued by investigator for this reason

the result. Prior clinical experience with the test in similar situations will assist this process.

We should select an appropriate frequency of determination and take samples at appropriate times in relation to dose. This should, as far as possible, take account of data already available. We must feel confident of the values of the results we eventually interpret. We should know what we might expect them to be and what the limitations are of the values with which we are provided. Normality and, therefore, abnormality are not absolute conditions. Our points of reference should be properly defined.

References

[1] Chuen Lee, P. and Hallsworth, P. Rapid viral diagnosis in perspective. *Brit. Med. J.*, **300**, 1413–18, 1990.
[2] Ciccolunghi, S.N., Fowler, P.D.L., and Chaudri, M.J. Interpretation of haematological and biochemical laboratory data in large scale-multicentre clinical trials. *J. Clin. Pharmacol.*, 303–12, 1979.
[3] Costongs, G.M.P.J., Janson, P.C.W., and Bas, B.M. Short-term and long-term intra-individual variation and critical differences of clinical chemistry laboratory parameters. *J. Clin. Chem. Clin. Biochem.*, **23**, 7–16, 1985.
[4] England, J.M., Chetty, M.C., Chadwick, R., *et al. Blood*, **46**, 321, 1975.

[5] England, J.M., Chetty, M.C., Chadwick, R., *et al.* An assessment of the Ortho ELT-8. *Clin. Lab. Haematol.*, **4**, 187, 1982.

[6] FDA. Minimal guidelines for detection of hepatotoxicity in early clinical trials of new drugs.

[7] Ford, H.C., Toolnath, R.J., Carter, J.M., *et al.* Mean platelet volume is increased in hyperthyroidism. *Am. J. Haematol.*, **27**, 190, 1988.

[8] Fraser, C.G. *Interpretation of Clinical Chemistry Laboratory Data*, Blackwell Scientific, Oxford, 1986.

[9] Grasbeck, R. *Reference Values in Laboratory Medicine, the Current State of the Art*, J. Wiley, Chichester, UK, 1981.

[10] Hardison, J.E. Sounding boards: to be complete. *N. Engl. J. Med.*, **300**, 193, 1979.

[11] Paulus, J.M. Platelet size in man. *Blood*, **46**, 321–6, 1975.

[12] Rose, M.S. Epitaph for the MCHC. *Brit. Med. J.*, **4**, 169, 1971.

[13] Skedzel, L.P., Barnett, R.N., and Platt, R. Medically useful criteria for analytical performance of laboratory tests. *Am. J. Clin. Pathol.*, **83**, 200–57, 1985.

.

12. Cancer Chemotherapy – Tumour Markers

J.G. McVie

Definition

A tumour marker has classically been a protein found in plasma/serum or in urine of cancer patients. Ideally, a tumour marker should be present in a concentration in direct proportion to the number of cancer cells in the body, but in reality this is rarely the case. The two tumour markers which have stood the test of time and are in regular use in patient management are alpha-feto-protein (AFP) and human chorionic gonadotrophin (HCG). From the names, it is clear that these two examples are not exclusive to cancers and neither is typical of only one form of cancer.

Choriocarcinoma is typified by a rise in the marker HCG (also used as a pregnancy test) after the foetus has aborted, so one could say that the first use of this tumour marker is in suggesting the diagnosis of mole or malignant mole. HCG is also found frequently in raised titres in serum in men with testicular teratoma, where it can be seen as a single marker or may be accompanied by AFP. AFP in turn can also be at raised levels in plasma in association with some liver tumours. Only in choriocarcinoma and teratoma have those two tumour markers been essential in patient management.

Application

The principal use of tumour markers is not so much to assist and diagnose (apart from the rare example of HCG and choriocarcinoma), but rather they are used to monitor response to therapy. Thus a young man with a swelling of his testis, thought to be malignant, should have AFP and HCG carried out before orchidectomy. Following orchidectomy, the tumour markers should be measured twice weekly for two or three weeks and, assuming that the swelling is a teratoma and is one of the common varieties which produce one or both of the markers, the behaviour of the markers will be indicative of the tumour bulk. If the tumour was localised to the testis and was therefore (by definition) cured by orchidectomy, the serum concentrations will fall to normal at a rate which indicates the half-life of the natural protein. Should the serum concentrations fall more slowly or rise, this represents a signal for further investigations and staging of the patient to detect either overt or microscopic metastases.

Fortunately, in patients with teratoma and choriocarcinoma, success rates with chemotherapy are spectacular and the response to cytotoxic drugs can be monitored in the same way as response to orchidectomy described above. The great benefit of these tumour markers is that they really do seem to reflect the bulk of the disease. Therefore, a normal concentration will generally indicate complete remission and a persistently normal level will indicate a probable cure. The converse is true in that a patient who is less than completely sensitive to cytotoxic drugs, and who will achieve a partial remission to first line choice of cytotoxic agents, will not undergo normalisation of serum markers and this is a useful signal for the therapist to switch to other non-cross-resistant drugs.

Other Markers

A host of cancer-associated antigens has been detected thanks to the revolution in immunology accompanying monoclonal antibody technology. Sadly, none of the agents is truly cancer specific, in the sense that AFP and HCG are for teratoma and choriocarcinoma. Perhaps the most useful apart from those two is acid phosphatase in the management of elderly men with prostate cancer metastasised to bone. However, not all bone metastases produce raised serum acid phosphatase concentrations, and the behaviour of serum concentrations is not always a good reflection of response to therapy nor prediction of long-term remission. (Cure in metastasised prostate cancer does not exist).

The most commonly used tumour marker is probably carcino-embryonic antigen, not because it is particularly useful, but because it is raised in a variety of common cancers, such as colon cancer, some breast cancers and pancreatic cancer. This antigen can be raised in serum to moderately high values in association with smoking, and so care must be taken in the interpretation of results.

Large studies with follow-up of patients with successfully resected colon cancer have shown that approximately one-half will produce carcino-embryonic antigen a few months before metastasis becomes obvious. As treatment of metastases in colon cancer, breast cancer or pancreas is far less successful than teratoma, these tumour marker rises have not been an indication for therapy; rather they indicate the need for extra alertness by the clinician. Numerous other antigens related to ovarian cancer, colon cancer and breast cancer are available and measurement kits are marketed with more or less extravagant claims; without exception they all have the same limitations as carcino-embryonic antigen.

New Markers

The discovery of oncogenes, and the fact that many of them code for growth factors or growth factor receptors, has opened up a new area of potential tumour markers. It is clear that some oncogenes, such as P53 mutation, are cancer specific. They need not always be present in all cancers, and it seems now that for colon cancer, breast cancer and bronchogenic carcinoma more than one oncogene is over expressed or mutated in some way in each cancer specimen. Nevertheless, the fact that these oncogenes frequently code for proteins which are detected on the membrane of cells means that they can be used as tumour cell markers. Some growth factor receptors are already used in oncology, such as the oestrogen receptor in breast cancer. This is of value in confirming malignant disease, giving some prognostic significance and predicting the likelihood of response to hormone intervention. The same may yet be true of other oncogenes presently being studied. The myc oncogene, for instance, is now clearly shown to be of value in predicting prognosis in neuroblastoma. The K-ras is specifically mutated at the twelfth amino acid in adenocarcinoma of the lung. The 30% of patients who have this mutation have a poorer prognosis than the rest of the population with the same histological type of cancer. Similarly the neu or C-erb oncogene predicts well for bulk of tumour in breast cancer. The future will see developments of a battery of tests and techniques for targeting these probes for imaging, and perhaps even for carrying therapeutic molecules to the cancer cells.

There is one other interesting development in tumour markers and this has to do with prediction of drug resistance in individual human tumours. Two examples are the enzyme topoisomerase and the P180 glycoprotein. Topoisomerase II has recently been identified as an enzyme located in the nucleus, responsible for DNA nicking, separating strands and religating. It is a target for some well-known cytotoxic agents such as etoposide, teniposide, doxorubicin and m-AMSA. Even more interesting is the finding of mutant forms of these enzymes in cell lines which have been proved to be resistant to the above classes of drugs. It means that, with a probe for the mutant enzyme, one will be able to scan tumours and mark patients unsuitable for certain drug therapy because it is known that the tumours are resistant. Alternatively, the probe might be used to follow the emergence of drug resistance in patients who are on conventional therapy involving those drugs. In this way these probes will be used as conventional tumour markers.

The phenomenon of multi-drug resistance (MDR) has been explored in a variety of cell lines from human tumours. If one such cell line is exposed continuously to low concentrations of a natural product, such as vincristine, doxorubicin or colchicine, the cell line will become resistant to that drug and to most other naturally occurring anti-tumour agents, including all the antibiotics and alkaloids. Coincident with this change is overexpression of the gene and overexpression at the cell membrane of P180 glycoprotein. It has been shown that this is a sophisticated pump protein which is long preserved in evolution and used for getting rid of a variety of noxious molecules of varying pharmacological characteristics. This pump can be blocked competitively by non-cytotoxic drugs, such as calcium channel agents, tetracycline or cyclosporin, and this could offer an important therapeutic tactic for overcoming this kind of drug resistance. Lately, overexpression of P-glycoprotein has been found in human tumours, both those not treated and those exposed to cytotoxic drugs, and therefore this laboratory model is now being seriously studied in the clinical situation. Monoclonal antibodies are available to the P-glycoprotein, and thus primary drug-resistant tumours can be signalled with simple application of monoclonal antibodies and appropriate therapeutic strategies can be evolved. Similarly, emergence of drug-resistant clones can be monitored and appropriate changes in drug treatment instituted.

Conclusion

There is no overall cancer test; there is no one pan-carcinoma tumour marker. The two useful markers AFP and HCG are unfortunately only useful for very rare tumours (teratoma and choriocarcinoma), and there is an urgent need for equally sensitive tumour markers for the common carcinomas. It is likely that a new generation of tumour markers will be found during oncogene research, and that they could be growth factor receptors, natural or mutated, mRNAs, enzymes or proteins located on tumour membrane or shed into the serum.

13. Anthracycline-Induced Cardiotoxicity and its Relevance in Cancer Treatment

C. Praga, F. Trave and A. Petroccione

Introduction

Anthracycline cardiotoxicity was first reported more than twenty years ago as an unexpected, late and fatal event in children successfully treated with daunorubicin for acute leukaemia and having reached complete remission.[12] Since then, cardiotoxicity has always been a matter of concern for the physician who uses daunorubicin (DNR), doxorubicin (DXR) or their most recent derivatives for the treatment of haematologic malignancies or solid tumours.

The clinical spectrum of anthracycline cardiotoxicity comprises early and late effects.[3] The early effects, which are observed after a single dose of the drug, are rare, transient and generally not life-threatening. They include mainly ECG changes and arrhythmias. The late effects, which are considerably more relevant from a clinical viewpoint, include cardiomyopathy or a congestive heart failure (CHF) directly related to myocyte injury.

DXR is the most extensively studied anthracycline as far as cardiotoxicity is concerned. The evaluation of clinical factors that enhance the risk of developing DXR cardiotoxicity was the object of two surveys carried out in Europe and in the USA[20] over ten years ago. The most important risk factor appears to be the cumulative dose of DXR; increasing this to over 550 mg/m^2 heightens the risk of CHF. Other potential risk factors include a 'prior mediastinal irradiation' of at least 2000 rad to the ventricles, age over 70 years and 'prior abnormal left ventricular function'.

A variety of methods for monitoring patients receiving DXR for the early detection of heart damage have been used. Careful questioning and examination of the patient during the course of treatment remain useful first steps in minimising the clinical impact of initial DXR cardiotoxicity. A decrease in the total electrocardiographic QRS voltage measured in the limb leads during DXR therapy was initially proposed as a means of predicting cardiotoxicity.[14] This parameter, however, was found to be an unreliable predictor of cardiac dysfunction by Henderson *et al.*[6] Two other non-invasive tests, systolic time intervals[6] and ejection fractions measured from the echocardiogram[5], have likewise proved to be insufficiently specific for practical patient management.

Radionuclide angiocardiography is currently the most promising non-invasive method of identifying patients likely to develop cardiotoxicity.[1] The

Table 13.1. Guidelines for monitoring patients receiving doxorubicin.[17]

- Perform baseline radionuclide angiocardiography at rest for calculation of the left ventricular ejection fraction (LVEF) prior to administration of a total dose of 100 mg/m^2 doxorubicin

I . *Patient with normal baseline LVEF ($\geq$50%)*
    A.   Perform the second study after 250 to 300 mg/m^2
    B.   Repeat study after 400 mg/m^2 in high-risk patients, or after 450 mg/m^2 in the absence of any known risk factor
    C.   Perform sequential studies thereafter prior to each dose
    D.   Discontinue doxorubicin therapy once functional criteria for cardiotoxicity develop, i.e., absolute decrease in LVEF $\geq$10% (EF units) associated with a decline to a level $\leq$50% (EF units)

II. *Patients with abnormal baseline LVEF ($<$50%)*
    A.   With baseline LVEF $\leq$30%, doxorubicin should not be started
    B.   In patients with LVEF $>$30% and $<$50%, sequential studies should be obtained *prior* to each dose
    C.   Discontinue doxorubicin with cardiotoxicity: absolute decrease in LVEF $\geq$10% (EF units) and/or final LVEF $\leq$30%

---

multiple gated imaging technique[21] may detect impaired cardiac function before irreversible changes occur, allowing such changes to be prevented by stopping DXR.

Finally, endomyocardial biopsy has proved useful in detecting pathological heart changes before clinical signs or symptoms develop. A pathological grading system, to score the degree of cardiac damage, has been developed by the Stanford group.[2] Patients with a score of 3+ are very likely to develop overt heart failure and should not receive more DXR. The invasive nature of this approach limits its use to investigations in specialised centres. In contrast, nuclear scans enjoy an increasing popularity both for investigational purposes and for cardiologic monitoring of individual patients treated with anthracyclines.

The largest experience in monitoring cardiac function in cancer patients using serial radionuclide angiocardiography has been acquired at Yale and Rochester Universities.[1] On the basis of their initial experience, these groups developed guideline criteria (*Table 13.1*) for cumulative dose-related scheduling of serial radionuclide angiocardiography and for discontinuing DXR administration. Their goal was to treat patients with DXR in such a way as to permit functional assessment of incipient cardiotoxicity prior to major clinical manifestations. Recommendations on both nuclear scan scheduling and termination of drug treatment are different in patients with normal and abnormal baseline left ventricular ejection fractions (LVEF).

Recently, Schwartz *et al.*[17] have analysed retrospectively a subset of 282 high-risk patients, selected from nearly 1500 cancer patients referred for LVEF monitoring over a seven-year period in both university and community hospitals. Clinical CHF occurred in 46 (16%) of these high-risk patients during the treatment period. The occurrence of CHF was compared in those patients whose management was concordant with proposed criteria (2/70) and in those whose management was not (44/212). Not only did the first group have a significantly lower incidence of CHF, but the two cases observed were also mild and not fatal. Multivariate analysis demonstrated a four-fold reduction in the incidence of CHF, independent of other clinical predictor variables in those patients whose management was concordant with the proposed guidelines.

These results, which might have important clinical implications because of their retrospective nature, suggest the advisability of a prospective trial to validate the guidelines further. In addition, treatment discontinuation according to precise guidelines might represent an important end point in clinical protocols for the assessment of new analogues or new cardioprotectors without exposing the patient to the serious risk of CHF.

Prevention of Cardiotoxicity

Several approaches have been suggested and applied to prevent cardiotoxicity from DXR and DNR.

The weekly administration of DXR does reduce the risk of cardiotoxicity, as well as that of other acute adverse effects.[19,23] However, this advantage has to be balanced against the need for more frequent injections of the drug which is inconvenient for patients and may expose them to a higher risk of extravasation.

Use of a continuous infusion to reduce the risk of cardiotoxicity is still a matter of debate, but it has always found strenuous support.[8]

The administration of 'protective agents' has been advocated on the basis of experimental studies, but clinic studies have only confirmed the value of ICRF–187 (see below).

Finally, the most important approach has been the development of less cardiotoxic anthracyclines.[24]

When a programme for the development of new anthracycline analogues was initiated in our laboratories, the reduction of cardiotoxicity was one of the major goals. *Figure 13.1* shows the general structure of anthracyclines as well as the molecular modifications that were made. The DXR and DNR analogues were largely studied in the 1980s, and are now available in the UK, with the exception of iodorubicin which is still an investigational drug. In the case of epirubicin, the only change is the epimerisation of the amino sugar in position 4'. This small configurational change has major pharmacokinetic and metabolic consequences.[22]

Epirubicin Cardiotoxicity

The preclinical profile of epirubicin (EPI), which shows lower cardiotoxicity at doses producing the same tumour responses as DXR, suggested that EPI might pose less cardiotoxic risk in humans. In the early clinical development of EPI, its therapeutic index was investigated and compared to that of DXR. On the basis of information from randomised studies, the lower cardiotoxicity of EPI at equiactive doses[9-16] was confirmed and it became available in the 1980s for the treatment of several tumour types.

The safety of EPI was assessed from a survey of 9144 patients treated with

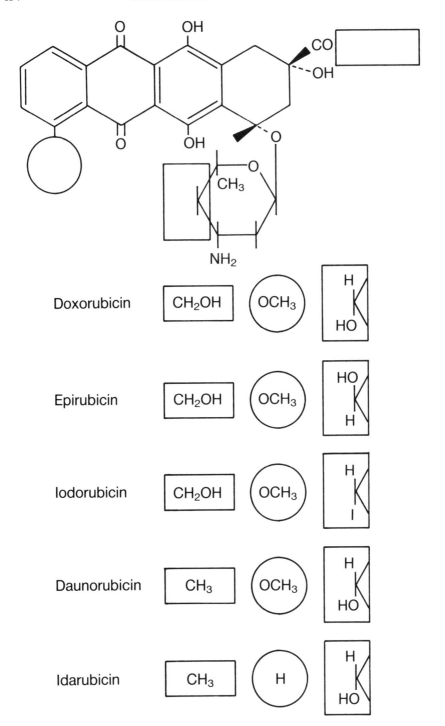

Figure 13.1. Chemical structure of antitumour anthracyclines related to doxorubicin.

Table 13.2. Epirubicin safety survey: patient and treatment characteristics.

	No. of cases	*Per cent*
Total	**9144**	**100.0**
Sex		
Male	1897	20.7
Female	7231	79.1
No data	16	0.2
Age		
<15	34	0.4
15–55	4658	50.9
>55	4381	47.9
No data	71	0.8
Geographic area		
Europe	5621	61.5
Australasia	798	8.6
Latin America	1689	18.5
Multinationals	1036	11.4
Tumour		
Breast		
Total	5633	61.6
Advanced	3943	43.1
Adjuvant	1690	18.5
Non-Breast		
Total	3511	38.4
G.I. tract	668	7.3
Lung	625	6.8
Gynaecological	688	7.5
Lymphomas	561	6.1
Others	969	10.5
Regimen		
EPI as single agent	2159	23.6
EPI in combination	6972	76.2
No data	13	0.2
Dose/Cycle		
Conventional dose: $\leq$90 mg/m^2	8041	87.9
High dose: >90 mg/m^2	1103	12.1
Previous mediastinal radiotherapy		
Yes	1693	18.5
No	7298	79.8
No data	153	1.7

the drug, alone or in combination, for a number of tumours in different geographical areas (*Table 13.2*). Breast cancer was the tumour most largely represented in this survey and explains the prevalence of female subjects. About half of the patients were over 55 years of age.

Administration of EPI, as is usual in cancer chemotherapy, has been in combination with other cytostatic drugs. Consequently, the safety profile indicated by this survey was more indicative of the toxicity of EPI-containing regimens than of that of EPI itself. EPI has been registered for clinical use at doses up to 90 mg/m^2/cycle. Therefore, all studies carried out with doses lower than, or equal to, 90 mg/m^2/cycle were identified as 'conventional dose studies' (CD), while investigational treatments employing epirubicin at doses above this threshold were classified as 'high-dose studies' (HD), irrespective of any combination with other cytostatic drugs. Finally, 18% of patients had received a previous mediastinal irradiation, a known risk factor for anthracycline cardiomyopathy.

The median cumulative dose (MCD) in the overall population was 300 mg/m^2, with a range from 11 to 2350 mg/m^2. Of the population surveyed, 1700 patients (18.2%) received a cumulative dose of EPI higher than 550 mg/m^2 (the maximum suggested cumulative dose of the established compound DXR), while only 127 patients were treated with a cumulative dose higher than 1000 mg/m^2.

Information on the most severe adverse events was obtained retrospectively from the case record forms of EPI-treated patients by means of a data-collecting sheet called 'safety abstract'. Apart from the data for patient, study and treatment identification, each safety abstract collated three areas of information:

- Severe unwanted events observed during treatment.
- Some risk factors for drug-related cardiotoxicity (total EPI cumulative dose; previous anthracycline chemotherapy; previous mediastinal radiotherapy).
- Reason for withdrawal from treatment.

Life-threatening infections, WHO grade 4 nausea/vomiting, WHO grade 4 mucositis[13], as well as symptomatic congestive heart failure (CHF), were unwanted events specifically requested by the safety abstract; their incidence in the total population was 1.91%, 1.70%, 0.34% and 0.71%, respectively. It should be emphasised that the role played by other cytostatic drugs given in combination with EPI is important as far as toxicity other than CHF is concerned. Cis-platinum, for instance, which was included in many of the protocols, frequently induces severe nausea and vomiting.

Symptomatic CHF was observed in 65 patients and was fatal in 14 of them (Table 13.3). The median cumulative dose in the CHF group was 660 mg/m^2 (range 89–1563 mg/m^2), which is more than twice that in the total population (300 mg/m^2). In 80% of the cases, CHF occurred during treatment and was a definite cause of withdrawal; in the remaining 20% it occurred during follow-up. Apart from the 65 cases of CHF, 125 other cardiac events were reported spontaneously in the safety abstract. Their exact incidence, seriousness and relationship to drug treatment could not be ascertained.

Systematic monitoring of left ventricular function was required by some protocols only. It is noteworthy, however, that impaired cardiac function (pathological reduction of the ventricular ejection fraction) was reported in at least 58 patients, and was the reason for withdrawal in two-thirds of them. The median cumulative dose of EPI in this group of patients was 560 mg/m^2, which was higher than that in the overall population (300 mg/m^2), but lower than that in the group with diagnosed CHF (660 mg/m^2). It is possible that the patients in this group would subsequently have suffered from symptomatic CHF.

Table 13.3. Epirubicin safety survey: unwanted cardiac events.

	Total		Definite reason for withdrawal		Fatal	
	No.	MCD*	No.	(%)	No.	(%)
Congestive heart failure (CHF)	65	660	52	80.0	14	21.5
Other cardiac events	125		79	63.2	12	9.8
Impaired cardiac function (non-CHF)	58	560	38	65.5	–	–
Arrhythmias only	27	360	17	63.0	2	7.4
Ischaemic disorders only	12	210	11	91.7	8	66.7
Mixed or not sufficiently specified	28	385	13	46.4	2	7.1

* MCD: median cumulative dose of EPI (mg/m^2).

The cumulative dose is the most important risk factor for the occurrence of CHF in a patient undergoing treatment with DXR. As expected in this large patient population treated with EPI, the probability of developing CHF increased with increasing cumulative dose (*Figure 13.2*). Logistic regression[4] of CHF on the cumulative dose was highly significant ($p<0.0001$). The risk of CHF is around 1% at a cumulative dose of 550 mg/m^2, and slowly approaches 5% at 1000 mg/m^2, increasing substantially beyond this dose.

Further analysis introducing potential risk factors has shown that treatment with high dose EPI per cycle is accompanied by a lower risk of CHF than treatment with conventional dose EPI per cycle. However, above a cumulative dose of 900–1000 mg/m^2, the probability of CHF increases more for HD EPI than for CD EPI. Mediastinal radiotherapy was highlighted by the analysis as a further risk factor ($p = 0.05$). Among other possible factors investigated, patients over 55 years of age were at higher risk of developing CHF, although statistical significance was not reached ($p = 0.08$).

Of previous retrospective surveys of DXR cardiotoxicity, that carried out by Von Hoff on 4018 patients[20] is the most similar to the present EPI survey in terms of sample size and characteristics of the population. In Von Hoff's study, however, the Kaplan–Mejer method[10] was used to estimate the probability of CHF. For comparative purposes, Kaplan–Mejer curves from both Von Hoff's DXR survey and the present EPI survey are shown in *Figure 13.3*. The shape of the two curves is similar. However, the inflexion of the curve occurs between 500 and 550 mg/m^2 for DXR and between 950 and 1000 mg/m^2 in the case of EPI. This historical comparison indicates that, by keeping the total dose of EPI at 950 mg/m^2, a level of CHF risk is accepted that is not higher than that associated with the standard cumulative dose of DXR.

The significance of the foregoing comparison must be assessed with respect to the effective dosage of the two drugs. It appears from these data that the cumulative dosages of DXR and EPI with respect to CHF approach a 1:2

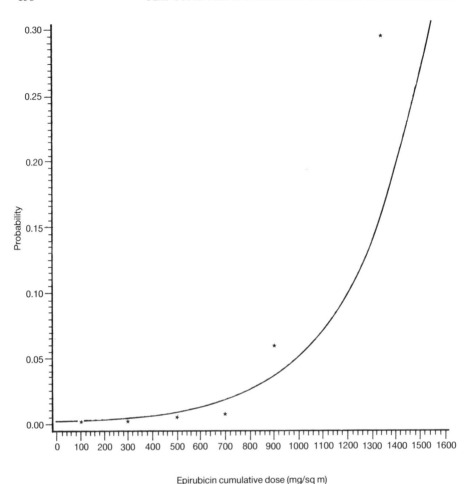

Figure 13.2. Logistic regression of the probability of congestive heart failure (CHF) on the cumulative dose of epirubicin (9144 cases). Regression parameters ($\alpha = -6.7718$; $\beta = 0.0038$) were highly significant ($p<0.0001$).

ratio. The doses of EPI generally required for clinical efficacy are in the range of 75–90 mg/m^2 and those of DXR in the range of 60–75 mg/m^2. The corresponding DXR/EPI efficacy dose ratio ranges from 1:1 to 1:1.5. Thus EPI is a less cardiotoxic analogue for conventional treatment with anthracyclines. However, a clinical problem still exists whenever high dose or prolonged anthracycline regimens may be of benefit and when dealing with patients who are at increased risk of developing cardiac toxicity.

Cardioprotection

ICRF-187 is the only agent that has been shown to confer in the clinic the cardioprotective properties observed in animal models[7]. It is the water

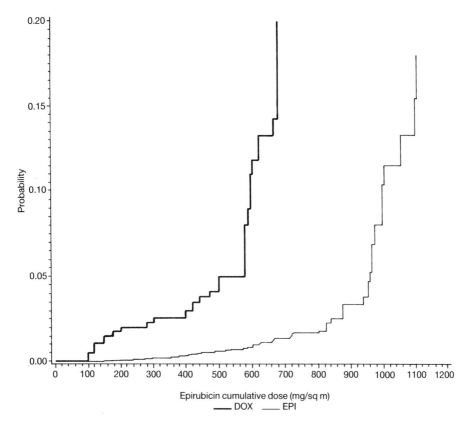

Figure 13.3. Cumulative probability of developing congestive heart failure (CHF) *versus* total cumulative dose. An historical comparison of descriptive Kaplan–Mejer curves for doxorubicin (after Von Hoff *et al.*[20]) and epirubicin (present safety survey).

soluble *D*-isomer of ICRF-159 or razoxane, extensively studied as an anti-tumour agent especially in the UK.

Probably because of its alkylating ability, ICRF-187 was also tested initially by the National Cancer Institute (NCI) for clinical antitumour activity, but the results were unsatisfactory. In contrast, a randomised trial in breast cancer, sponsored by the NCI and conducted at New York University, confirmed its protective effect against DXR-induced cardiac toxicity.[18] A simple experimental design was used. One group received FDC, a standard DXR-containing combination for the treatment of advanced breast cancer. Another group received the same regimen preceded by the administration of ICRF-187.

There was no predetermined cumulative dose at which DXR could be discontinued. Patients were withdrawn from the study when cardiac toxicity developed or the cancer progressed. The cardiological criteria for discontinuing treatment were clinical signs of congestive heart failure, a fall in the resting LVEF to less than 45% or a fall from baseline of 20% or more, and a biopsy graded 2 or over.

Table 13.4. ICRF-187/doxorubicin cardioprotection trial: comparison of cardiac toxicity between two groups receiving chemotherapy with and without ICRF-187.[18]

	FDC	FDC/ICRF-187	P (t test)
Clinical cardiotoxicity	11/45	2/47	0.02
Endomyocardial biopsy			
Biopsy score ≥2	5/13	0/13	0.03
Left ventricular ejection fraction			
(nuclear scan)			
Basal LVEF (%)	66.1	63.6	–
Mean fall (%) from base line			
at the DXR cumulative dose of:			
250–399 mg/m^2	6.6	1.6	0.02
400–499 mg/m^2	15.4	1.4	<0.001
500–599 mg/m^2	15.8	3.0	0.003

The antitumour response rates (CR-PR), as well as the time to progression, were similar in the two groups and, although myelosuppression was slightly greater in the ICRF group, the incidence of fever, infections and deaths due to toxicity did not differ between the two groups.

The evaluation of cardiac toxicity by clinical examination, endomyocardial biopsy or by measurement of the left ventricular ejection fraction using multigated nuclear scans showed a highly significant difference between the groups (*Table 13.4*). Below a DXR cumulative dose of 400 mg/m^2, the mean fall in the LVEF was quite small, but ICRF-187 clearly afforded a significant cardioprotection. The differences between the two groups increased at higher DXR cumulative doses.

According to the authors of this study, ICRF-187 is a promising cardio-protector and is now under clinical development in both the USA and Europe.

Conclusion

Cardiotoxicity is an important limiting factor in anthracycline therapy, but probably less so than the occurrence of drug-resistance.[11] However, experience with anthracycline cardiotoxicity illustrates the importance of a reliable clinical method of monitoring specific drug toxicity in the process of drug development.

References

[1] Alexander, J., Dainiak, N., Berger, H.J., Goldman, L., Johnstone, D., Reduto, L., Duffy, T., Schwartz, P., Gottschalk, A., and Zaret, B.L. Serial assessment of doxorubicin cardiotoxicity with quantitative radionuclide angiocardiography. *New Eng. J. Med.*, **300**, 278–83, 1979.
[2] Billingham, M.E., Mason, J.W., Bristow, M.R., and Daniels, J.R. Anthra-

cycline cardiomyopathy monitored by morphologic changes. *Cancer Treatment Rep.*, **62**, 865–72, 1978.

[3] Bristow, M.R., Billingham, M.E., Mason, J.W., and Daniels, J.R. Clinical spectrum of anthracycline antibiotic cardiotoxicity. *Cancer Treatment Rep.*, **62**, 873–9, 1978.

[4] Cox, D.R. The linear logistic model. In *The Analysis of Binary Data*, M.S. Bartlett and D.R. Cox (eds), Chapman and Hall, London, pp 14–29, 1970.

[5] Ewy, G.A., Jones, S.E., Friedman, M.J., Gaines, J., and Cruze, D. Non-invasive cardiac evaluation of patients receiving adriamycin. *Cancer Treatment Rep.*, **62**, 915, 1978.

[6] Henderson, J.C., Sloss, L.J., Jaffe, N., Blum, R.H., and Frei, E. III. Serial studies of cardiac function in patients receiving adriamycin. *Cancer Treatment Rep.*, **62**, 923, 1978.

[7] Herman, E. and Ferrans, V.J. Pre-treatment with ICRF-187 provides long-lasting protection against chronic daunorubicin cardiotoxicity in rabbits. *Cancer Chemother. Pharmacol.*, **16**, 102–106, 1986.

[8] Hortobagyi, G.N., Frye, D., Buzdar, A.U., Ewer, M.S., Fraschini, G., Hug, V., Ames, F., Montague, E., Carrasco, C.H., Mackay, B., and Benjamin, R.S. Decreased cardiotoxicity of doxorubicin administered by continuous intravenous infusion in combination chemotherapy for metastatic breast carcinoma. *Cancer*, **63**, 37–45, 1989.

[9] Jain, K.K., Casper, E.S., Geller, N.L., *et al.* A prospective randomised comparison of epirubicin and doxorubicin in patients with advanced breast cancer. *J. Clin. Oncology*, **3**, 818–26, 1985.

[10] Kaplan, E.L. and Mejer, P. Non-parametric estimation from incomplete observations. *J. Am. Stat. Ass.*, **53**, 457–81, 1958.

[11] Kaye, S. and Merry, S. Tumour cell resistance to anthracyclines: a review. *Cancer Chemother. Pharmacol.*, **14**, 96–103, 1985.

[12] Macrez, C., Marneffe-Lebrequier, H., Ripault, J., Clauvel, J.P., Jacquillat, C., and Weil, M. Cardiac complications observed during treatment with rubidomycin. *Patholog. Biolog.*, **15**, 949–54, 1967.

[13] Miller, A.B., Hoogstraten, B., Staquet, M., and Winkler, A. Reporting results of cancer treatment. *Cancer*, **47**, 207–14, 1981.

[14] Minow, R.A., Benjamin, R.S., Lee, E.T., and Gottlieb, J.A. QRS voltage change with adriamycin administration. *Cancer Treatment Rep.*, **62**, 931, 1978.

[15] Praga, C., Beretta, G., Vigo, P.L., Lenaz, G.R., Pollini, C., Bonadonna, G., Canetta, R., Castellani, R., Villa, E., Gallagher, C.G., von Melchner, H., Hayat, M., Ribaud, P., de Wasch, G., Mattsson, W., Heinz, R., Waldner, R., Kolaric, K., Buehner, R., Ten Bokkel-Huyninck, W., Perevodchikova, N.I., Manziuk, L.A., Senn, H.J., and Mayr, A.C. Adriamycin cardiotoxicity: a survey of 1273 patients. *Cancer Treatment Rep.*, **63**, 827–34, 1979.

[16] Robert, J., Cersosimo, J. and Waun Ki Hong. Epirubicin: a review of the pharmacology, clinical activity and adverse effects of an adriamycin analogue. *J. Clin. Oncology*, **3**, 425–39, 1986.

[17] Schwartz, R.G., McKenzie, W.B., Alexander, J., Sager, P., Manatunga, A., Schwartz, P.E., Berger, H.J., Setaro, J., Surkin, L., Wackers, F.J., and Zaret, B.L. Congestive heart failure and left ventricular dysfunction complicating doxorubicin therapy. *Am. J. Med.*, **82**, 1109–18, 1987.

[18] Speyer, J., Green, M., Kramer, E., *et al*. Protective effects of bispiper-azinedione ICRF-187 against doxorubicin-induced cardiotoxicity in women with advanced breast cancer. *New Eng. J. Med.*, **319**, 745–52, 1988.

[19] Torti, F.M., Bristow, M.R., Howes, A.E., Aston, D., Stockdale, F.E., Carter, S.K., Kohler, M., Brown, B.W., and Billingham, M.E. Reduced cardiotoxicity of doxorubicin delivered on a weekly schedule: assessment by endomyocardial biopsy. *Ann. Int. Med.*, **99**, 745–9, 1983.

[20] Von Hoff, D.D., Layard, M.W., Basa, P., Davis, H.L., Von Hoff, A.L., Rozencweig, M., and Muggia, F.M. Risk factors for doxorubicin-induced congestive heart failure. *Ann. Int. Med.*, **91**, 710–17, 1979.

[21] Wackers, F.J., Berger, H.J., Johnstone, D.E., *et al*. Multiple-gated cardiac blood pool imaging for left ventricular ejection fraction: validation of the technique and assessment of variability. *Am. J. Cardiol.*, **43**, 1159–64, 1979.

[22] Weenen, H., Van Maanen, J.M.S., De Planque, M.M., McVie, J.G., and Pinedo, H.M. Metabolism of 4'-modified analogues of doxorubicin. Unique glucuronidation pathway for 4'-epi-doxorubicin. *Eur. J. Clin. Oncology*, **7**, 919–26, 1984.

[23] Weiss, A.J., Metter, G.E., Fletcher, W.S., Wilson, W.L., Grace, T.B., and Ramirez, G. Studies on adriamycin using a weekly regimen demonstrating its clinical effectiveness and lack of cardiac toxicity. *Cancer Treatment Rep.*, **60**, 813–22, 1976.

[24] Young, R.C., Ozols, R.F., and Myers, C.E. The anthracycline antineoplastic drugs. *New Eng. J. Med.*, **305**, 139–53, 1981.

14. Markers of Drug Allergy

L.J.F. Youlten

Introduction

This review is limited to allergic drug reactions in the Type I or immediate hypersensitivity category, and to those reactions whose clinical features mimic such reactions and are therefore classified as 'pseudo-allergic' or 'anaphylactoid'. True anaphylactic hypersensitivity is most often mediated by IgE. In its most familiar form, it is typified by acute generalised reactions, occasionally fatal, to bee or wasp venom, or, more commonly, to inhalant or ingestant allergens such as dust mite, pollen or animal proteins, or, more rarely, food proteins or other macromolecules.

Anaphylaxis is a relatively uncommon form of drug hypersensitivity, but the serious consequences of failing to recognise it, or to follow up survivors with appropriate investigation and advice, justify concentrating on it in this review to the exclusion of the other forms of drug allergy which have been described. These include examples of all the Types I–IV of hypersensitivity reaction as described by Gell and Coombs.

Type I Hypersensitivity

A brief account of the classic Type I hypersensitivity, exemplified by bee venom allergy, follows:

- Induction of sensitivity: following one or more stings (which involve up to 50µg of foreign protein, mainly enzymes, being injected into the skin), some individuals respond by producing high titres of IgE specifically directed towards one or more of the protein antigens in the venom.
- This IgE becomes attached to high and low affinity receptor sites on mast cells, blood basophils, platelets and possibly other cells/tissues.
- If specific IgE is still present on these potentially mediator-releasing cells at the time of a subsequent sting, venom antigens can trigger massive release of a potent mixture of pre-formed and newly synthesised inflammatory mediators, including histamine, prostaglandins and leukotrienes.
- The released mediators, by interaction with receptors on target tissues, including vascular, bronchial or intestinal smooth muscle, the heart, etc., produce local and/or generalised effects. The exact outcome of these

depends, not only on the types and amounts of mediators released, but also on the target organ sensitivity of the victim at the time of the sting.

There are other (non-IgE) mechanisms which can lead to an identical result, including direct effects on mediator-releasing cells, e.g. by codeine phosphate, or by other immunological pathways, e.g. by antigen/IgG reactions, activating the complement pathway to produce anaphylatoxins, with direct and/or indirect (via mast cell activation) effects.

In the case of drugs which are themselves proteins, it is not surprising that IgE-mediated hypersensitivity can occur. For proteins and other potentially antigenic molecules introduced into man as novel drugs, the question of allergenicity, and also of immunogenicity in general, is one which has major implications, for both safety and sustained efficacy. Drugs of this type may be antigenically similar to naturally occurring environmental allergens, and patients may in these circumstances react adversely to the first exposure.

This is analogous to the situation in beekeepers, a few of whom get sensitised to venom by inhalation of fine venom dust, rather than the more usual injected (sting) route, and theoretically can react to their first sting with anaphylaxis. Similarly, horse serum or streptokinase used therapeutically may elicit hypersensitivity responses on first administration to individuals sensitised by, in the first case, inhalation or, in the second, by streptococcal infection. Although it is moderately immunogenic, animal-based insulin causes problems relatively rarely, possibly because of a state of immunological tolerance induced by daily injections. Restarting insulin after a period without it may carry an increased likelihood of precipitating such reactions.

When drugs which are not macromolecules, and not therefore intrinsically likely to act as antigens, provoke apparent anaphylaxis, the mechanisms involved may be somewhat different. In some instances, the drug itself, or a metabolite, can form a covalent linkage with a soluble protein or other macromolecule. In these circumstances, the drug or metabolite is said to be acting as a 'hapten'. The hapten–protein complex is then recognised as a foreign protein by the immune system, and antibodies, including in some individuals IgE, directed against the hapten conjugate are produced. In some cases, these antibodies (generally of the IgG class) will specifically bind the unconjugated hapten and, when this is a drug, it can form the basis of immunoassay, for which animals or isolated lymphocytes produce the highly specific antisera.

Apart from hapten formation, there appears to be another pathway to anaphylaxis, typified by aspirin hypersensitivity, in which vulnerable individuals suffer the effects of activation of mast cells and other mediator sources by mechanisms independent of antibody production.

Almost any drug can, in occasional individuals, cause anaphylaxis and, when this is a very rare occurrence in the subject, the type of mechanism involved may never be known. Often, all that is done in practice is to warn survivors of such reactions to avoid further exposure to the source or closely related agents.

Some drug classes, however, are recognised as being more likely than others to cause such potentially serious reactions. The remainder of this review deals briefly with several such drug classes involving widely used drugs, and illustrates some of the approaches which have been used to elucidate the nature of the reactions, to identify patients at risk and to reassure them and their doctors that proposed alternatives are safe.

Recognition

How can an anaphylactic or anaphylactoid reaction be recognised and differentiated from other acute reactions such as vasovagal attacks, hypoglycaemia, epilepsy, etc.? This process is not always easy, but the most helpful factor is the history, either from the patient, a witness or a doctor. Clinical features pointing strongly to anaphylaxis are itch, flush, weals and angioedema, voice change, stridor, wheeze and dyspnoea. Other features often present, but also seen in other acute reactions, include tachycardia and other arrhythmias, hypotension, sudden loss of consciousness and feeling of doom. Rarely, gastrointestinal or genito-urinary manifestations can be prominent features of anaphylaxis. A prompt clinical response to adrenaline injection can be a helpful supporting feature in cases of doubt.

Investigation

Attempts to measure plasma or urine inflammatory mediators or their metabolites, while theoretically helpful, are beset by technical problems and, given the short half-life of these mediators, the limited access to assays, the problems with artefacts or with baseline measurements, they have not proved particularly useful. Recently, however, Schwartz[7] in the USA has identified a specific mast cell derived tryptase which can be assayed in secretions or in plasma, and which remains detectable for some hours after reactions. An assay (Pharmacia Tryptase RIACT) for this mast cell activation marker is now commercially available, and may turn out to be of more practical use in the differentiation of anaphylactic–anaphylactoid reactions from other reactions than in histamine or methyl histamine assays.

Once a drug reaction has been categorised as anaphylactic–anaphylactoid, it is imperative, wherever possible, to identify the cause. In the case of drug allergy of this type, advice about avoidance should follow, and it is also necessary to monitor the patient's sensitivity by some reliable technique. The principles involved will be illustrated by reference to three commonly used drug groups, with features which exemplify the problems of this aspect of patient evaluation. These are: penicillin and other beta-lactam antibiotics; aspirin and other non-steroid anti-inflammatory drugs; and muscle relaxants and other drugs used in general anaesthesia.

Penicillin Allergy

This condition is among the most common to be claimed by patients, and is undoubtedly over-diagnosed. The consequences of mismanagement are potentially lethal, however, and the easy option is to take seriously any claim of past penicillin reactions and to avoid penicillins thereafter for life. Such a policy does deprive many patients of what can well be a safe, effective and cheap form of treatment. A great deal of attention has been given, therefore, to devising reliable tests of penicillin sensitivity, which should ideally be (but rarely are in practice) applicable to all patients with a past history of adverse reactions with clinical features consistent with anaphylaxis.

The mechanisms of immediate hypersensitivity reactions to penicillins are relatively well understood, although the situation is a complex one. Beta-lactam antibiotics such as penicillin may become immunogenic either before administration, for example by polymer formation, or after administration, as by conjugation with plasma or other proteins. Because of cross-reactivity of chemically similar molecules, the demonstration of skin test positive reactions to, or *in vitro* specific IgE directed against, a particular penicillin derivative is not any guarantee that this is the derivative responsible for sensitisation and/or elicitation of reactions. For purposes of clinical management, however, it seems reasonable to take an empirical approach to the problem, based on extensive studies of patients subsequently treated with penicillin.

One such study, from a group at the Johns Hopkins School of Medicine, studied nearly four thousand patients attending a sexually transmitted disease clinic in Baltimore.[1] The majority had no convincing history of prior reaction, and in this group a very small proportion of those with negative skin tests had some sort of systemic reaction to dosing with penicillin; less than one-quarter of these reactions, however, were considered to fall in the category of 'probably IgE-mediated'. When the history of a prior reaction was positive, but the nature of the reaction was not suggestive of anaphylaxis, positive skin tests were seen in only 2–6%, and reactions in 3–8% of the negative reactors, with less than 1% experiencing apparently IgE-mediated reactions. The picture began to change in those patients whose reaction suggested an anaphylactic mechanism, without full-blown clinical features, i.e. those who reported urticaria as the main feature of their reactions. Of these subjects, 17% had positive skin tests, and 11% of the negative skin test group had a generalised reaction to penicillin which, in more than half the cases, appeared to be IgE-dependent.

When the history was unequivocally that of anaphylaxis, five of a group of sixteen patients had positive skin tests, and two of nine with negative tests had generalised reactions, one of which was considered IgE-mediated. Thus, clinical history appeared to be an important consideration.

The reliability of skin testing has been clearly shown to depend on the nature of the reagents used. The predominant, so called major, antigenic determinant is the benzylpenicilloyl moiety (BPO), and a synthetic conjugate of this (penicilloyl polylysine) identifies 35–70% of patients with penicillin allergy. Some other patients react to penicillin-G itself, but it is only by also including the minor determinants, in particular penilloate and penicilloate, that skin testing with negative results becomes sufficiently reliable an indicator of absence of life-threatening sensitivity. The natural history of penicillin sensitivity, as elucidated by skin testing, is that, while a few patients can sustain their sensitivity for more than ten years without exposure to the antibiotic, the majority (78%) will lose their sensitivity with time. This was seen in a study in which most patients with a positive history were skin test positive when tested within a year of their reaction.[8] Current *in vitro* tests seem more likely to give false negative results than skin testing, which is therefore the most appropriate technique for investigating a patient's current status in relation to penicillin allergy. Attempts have been made to validate similar techniques for other antibiotics, including modified penicillin, cepha-losporin (both of which have a high level of cross reactivity with penicillin), and other antibiotics. Reagents for performing such tests are not available generally in a standardised form and, in spite of the clear results with penicillin allergy skin tests, the essential minor determinant reagents have still not been licensed for use in the USA or UK. They are thus only available on a 'named patient' basis and, in practice, it is currently easier to adopt the stratagem of finding alternative antibiotics for all patients with a history suggesting penicillin anaphylaxis, and performing desensitisation in hospital for such patients who have clinically pressing indications for penicillin treatment.

Aspirin and NSAID Hypersensitivity

In contrast with penicillin sensitivity, there is, in the great majority of patients with aspirin hypersensitivity, no evidence whatsoever of IgE, or any other immunoglobulin, being involved. There is a preponderance of females, and atopy does not seem to be a risk factor. Several features of this condition are distinctive, and some of them support a non-immunological or 'pseudo-allergic' mechanism. The condition is often apparent as a trigger factor for urticaria, late-onset asthma or rhino-sinusitis. Here it may be one among many exacerbating factors, where avoidance does not alleviate the clinical problem and development does not depend on prior exposure.

Cross-reactivity occurs to other NSAIDs whose chemical structures may vary, but which share the pharmacological property of being cyclo-oxygenase inhibitors.[6] No skin test or *in vitro* test has been shown to be useful in confirming or excluding aspirin sensitivity, and the only tests which carry a high degree of accuracy in diagnosing this condition are oral or inhaled provocation challenges. These, of course, require a cautious approach to avoid hazard to the patient, but the confirmation rate of histories of previous reaction to these drugs is high, unlike penicillin allergy. This is, perhaps, because the sensitivity, once established, does not wane spontaneously. A number of investigators have attempted to identify biochemical abnormalities in such patients which would help elucidate the mechanism of reactions and confirm sensitivity without the need for provocation tests. The cross-reactivity seen in such patients, which is matched by a cross-desensitisation, may be a useful feature for testing the potential of new anti-inflammatory drugs which could be safely tolerated by an aspirin-sensitive patient. This would be a possible benefit to justify cautious testing of new compounds in aspirin-sensitive patients.

Among the mechanisms which have been proposed to account for the phenomena of aspirin-sensitive asthma and urticaria are:

- Diversion of arachidonate down lipoxygenase pathways to produce more leukotrienes.
- Abnormalities of platelet response to these drugs.
- Displacement of inflammatory prostaglandins from plasma protein-binding sites by the drug.

Neuromuscular Blocking Drugs

These drugs rarely (approximately 1 per 5000 to 1 per 8000 exposures) cause anaphylactic–anaphylactoid reactions which, occurring in unconscious patients who have also received other i.v. drugs, may pose particular problems in recognition and management. Diagnostic indicators such as pruritus, flushing and even urticaria may be overlooked or discounted on the grounds that many drugs in this category have histamine-releasing properties. The clinical presentation is therefore either bronchospasm, with difficulty in inflating the lungs, or arterial hypotension. The differential diagnosis from other anaesthetic emergencies may be difficult, and improvement in response to adrenaline may be a helpful diagnostic factor. These reactions are, by their nature, always observed by a doctor, unlike the majority of aspirin or penicillin reactions, and therefore might form a useful group in which to validate confirmatory tests of the nature of the reaction, such as the tryptase test mentioned above.

Like aspirin sensitivity, this type of reaction does not depend on prior exposure to the drug concerned, often occurring during the patient's first general anaesthetic. Another similarity is that females predominate among the cases recorded. In other ways, however, there are obvious differences between this type of reaction and aspirin sensitivity. Cross-reactivity is limited and does not depend on pharmacological mode of action, and skin testing with the drugs themselves at appropriate concentrations is highly accurate in identifying the drug responsible and in excluding other drugs given at the same time. Furthermore, there is evidence both from passive transfer of serum (PK testing) and from *in vitro* techniques, such as RAST with appropriate solid phase drug conjugates[2,4], that these reactions are mediated by a specific IgE, although atopy *per se* is not a strong risk factor.

It remains a mystery as to how patients become sensitised without previous exposure. One theory is that it is molecules with two quaternary ammonium groups separated by a certain critical distance that are responsible, and that it is some other compound sharing this structural feature with one or more neuromuscular blocking drugs which is responsible for sensitisation, without itself precipitating any reactions. No direct evidence in favour of this hypothesis has been provided yet, and other explanations may have to be sought.

In practice, skin testing with appropriate concentrations of the different neuromuscular blocking drugs and anaesthetic induction agents is a most accurate method of identifying which drug was responsible for a reaction, and which alternatives should also be avoided in future anaesthetics.[3] The test requires no specialised techniques other than skin-prick testing, which can be learnt in a few minutes.[5] The answer is available also within minutes, and the test can be carried out with any available drugs which might be under consideration as safe alternatives. *In vitro* testing is at present not validated to the same extent, takes days to arrange, is relatively expensive, and is only available for a few drugs, namely suxamethonium, alcuronium and thiopentone. Much more work on the specificity and accuracy of such RAST tests will need to be done before they can rival skin testing as the 'gold standard' in this area of drug allergy.

Miscellaneous

There are other drug groups well recognised as carrying a higher than average risk of anaphylaxis. For some of these, such as the hyposensitising vaccines, the mechanism is obvious, although unknown factors may contribute to intermittent and therefore unpredictable sensitivity to such reactions. In other cases, such as plasma expanders and radiological contrast mediators, other mechanisms may be involved, such as complement activation, or hypertonic effects on mediator-releasing cells.

Conclusion

When assessing the potential to cause anaphylaxis of new compounds, the available information on other drugs in the same therapeutic class may sometimes suggest appropriate methods of evaluation. Skin testing, provocation testing or *in vitro* or *ex vivo* tests (such as basophil mediator release, platelet reactivity or complement studies) in patients with well-authenticated current hypersensitivity may in the end be the most helpful way of assessing the likelihood of cross-reactivity with existing drugs in this population of patients. It should be remembered, however, that more than one mechanism of activation can lead to anaphylaxis.

All doctors, but especially those administering drugs by injection, should be alert to the possibility of acute drug-induced anaphylaxis and aware of the importance of rapid diagnosis and appropriate treatment. They should not forget the responsibility of following up such patients and advising them how best to avoid future, potentially fatal, reactions to drugs.

References

[1] Adkinson, N.F. Risk factors for drug allergy. *J. Allergy Clin. Immunol.*, **74**, 567–72, 1984.

[2] Baldo, B.A. and Fisher, M. Substituted ammonium ions as allergenic determinants in drug allergy. *Nature*, **306**, 262–4, 1983.

[3] Fisher, M.McD. The diagnosis of acute anaphylactoid reactions to anaesthetic drugs. *Anaesth. Intens. Care*, **9**, 235–41, 1981.

[4] Harle, D., Baldo, B., and Fisher, M. Detection of IgE antibodies to suxamethonium after anaphylactoid reactions during anaesthesia. *Lancet*, **1**, 930–2, 1984.

[5] Leynadier, F., Sansarricq, M., Didier, J.M., and Dry, J. Prick tests in the diagnosis of anaphylaxis to general anaesthetics. *Br. J. Anaesth.*, **59**, 683–9, 1987.

[6] Mathison, D.A. and Stevenson, D.D. Hypersensitivity to non-steroidal anti-inflammatory drugs: indications and methods for oral challenge. *J. Allergy Clin. Immunol.*, **64**, 669–74, 1979.

[7] Schwartz, L.B., Metcalfe, D.D., Miller, J.S., Earl, H., and Sullivan, T. Tryptase levels as an indicator of mast cell activation in systemic anaphylaxis and mastocytosis. *New Eng. J. Med.*, **316**, 1622–6, 1987.

[8] Sullivan, T.J., Wedner, H.J., Shatz, G.S., Yecies, L.D., and Parker, C.W. Skin testing to detect penicillin allergy. *J. Allergy Clin. Immunol.*, **68**, 171–80, 1981.

15. Gastrointestinal Methodology for the Evaluation of Drug Effects in Man

P. Demol and T.R. Weihrauch

Introduction

'All things are a poison and none is without poison, only the dose makes that a thing is no poison' (Paracelsus, 1493–1541).

To prove the efficacy and safety of a drug in the treatment of a disease requires adequate and well-controlled studies. It is necessary, however, not only to show that the drug works, but also to determine the optimal dose and dose interval in which the drug should be used, as well as the optimal duration of therapy. In carefully designed therapeutic dose–response trials, this basic scientific demand can be achieved. Hereby the range from the minimal effective dose to the maximal therapeutic and well-tolerated dose can be assessed, and as a result the optimal dose range and dosage regimen can be defined.

Therapeutic dose finding trials, mostly carried out in the early phase of clinical drug development, need careful planning and biometric design. Whenever ethically possible, they should be carried out with placebo control and should compare at least two or, even better, three fixed doses. Individual dose titration should be avoided. Furthermore, the effectiveness of a drug should be supported by more than one well-controlled trial and performed by independent investigators in order to demonstrate the reproducibility of the results.[13]

Meaningful pharmacodynamic studies can be performed in healthy volunteers, provided that a method with a high predictability for the desired therapeutic effect is available (e.g. measurement of gastric acid secretion and its inhibition by a drug, like an H_2-receptor antagonist, or of oesophageal motility by manometry, which allows assessment of the efficacy of prokinetic or spasmolytic compounds). While careful clinical pharmacological dose–response studies have been carried out in man since the early 1970s, the situation is less clear for therapeutic clinical trials in gastrointestinal therapy. In fact, only during the past few years have different doses of an investigational drug been compared within one study.

For the evaluation of new drugs, new indications or new dosage regimens of known compounds in gastrointestinal therapy, a number of methods are

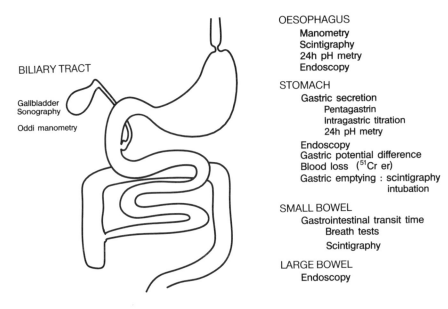

BILIARY TRACT

Gallbladder
Sonography

Oddi manometry

OESOPHAGUS
Manometry
Scintigraphy
24h pH metry
Endoscopy

STOMACH
Gastric secretion
Pentagastrin
Intragastric titration
24h pH metry
Endoscopy
Gastric potential difference
Blood loss (^{51}Cr er)
Gastric emptying : scintigraphy
intubation

SMALL BOWEL
Gastrointestinal transit time
Breath tests
Scintigraphy

LARGE BOWEL
Endoscopy

Figure 15.1. The most useful techniques for the evaluation of drug effects at the different levels of the digestive tract.

available which yield accurate and reproducible data *(Figure 15.1)*. These methods are described briefly and examples for dose–response studies are given.

Oesophagus

Oesophageal Manometry

Oesophageal manometry has become an established procedure for drug evaluation in man. With this method, the effect of drugs on smooth muscle in man can be investigated. Because of the direct accessibility of the oeso-phagus, the investigation is technically easy to perform and is well tolerated by the patient. A detailed description of this method is given elsewhere.[8,47]

Oesophageal manometry gives accurate and reproducible data of drug effects on lower oesophageal sphincter pressure (LOSP) and peristaltic contractions. Numerous acute single dose–response studies have been per-formed in healthy volunteers as well as in patients. Because its value for drug studies has been well established during the past decade, the term 'oeso-phageal pharmacomanometry' was proposed for this method.[48] Dose–response studies have been carried out using oesophageal pharmacomanome-try for prokinetic and spasmolytic compounds. The prokinetic compounds which have been studied in healthy volunteers and in patients with gastro-oesophageal reflux are metoclopramide, domperidone and cisa-pride.[10,17,25,39,49] The lower oesophageal sphincter pressure (LOSP) is increased by increasing doses of these drugs in a dose-dependent manner.

From the pharmacomanometric study of Stanciu and Bennett[39], a new pathophysiological conclusion could be drawn and this was important for the treatment of patients with reflux oesophagitis. In patients with severe disease, i.e. a significantly decreased lower oesophageal sphincter pressure, metoclopramide increased the sphincter tone only moderately while, in patients with an intact function, the increase was two- to three-fold. Recently it was shown (by oesophageal pharmacomanometry) that prostaglandin E1 and E2 analogues do not have a negative effect on oesophageal motility as was assumed from animal studies. On the contrary, in man, prostaglandin analogues increase LOSP dose–dependently in doses which are used for ulcer treatment.[3] This result is of importance in the treatment of peptic ulcer disease with regard to drug safety. Furthermore, it may make these prostaglandins useful in reflux oesophagitis and early therapeutic results confirm this observation.[37] This example shows how a myth, induced by an animal experiment which was obviously not adequate and/or was irrelevant for the therapy in man, can be corrected by well-designed and well-controlled clinical pharmacological and therapeutic studies.

Oesophageal pharmacomanometry has contributed significantly to the elucidation of the pathogenesis of primary oesophageal motility disorders, e.g. diffuse oesophageal spasm (DOS) and achalasia, as well as their treatment. It can be shown that nitrates, calcium antagonists and β_2-antagonists influence abnormal motility patterns. For calcium antagonists of the dihydropyridine type (e.g. nifedipine), a dose-dependent effect on oesophageal motility in healthy volunteers has been demonstrated.[2]

Endoscopy

Endoscopic examinations are of great importance for dose–response studies in patients with reflux oesophagitis and only recently have such studies with comparison of different doses become available. For the quantitative assessment of therapeutic improvement by scoring, a system for the severity of the lesions is used. Until now, only very few true dose–response studies have been carried out, but Kaul and others[23] compared the effect of two dose regimens of cimetidine (400 mg bid. and 400 mg qid.) with placebo and found equally significant positive effects with both regimens after 6 and 12 weeks. However, placebo-controlled dose–response studies comparing different doses in the same dose regimen are needed.

pH-Metry

Twenty-four-hour pH-metry for the assessment of gastro-oesophageal reflux and the effect of drugs is being used increasingly. Portable instruments and computer-assisted evaluation have improved the value of the method significantly. Reproducibility is fairly good, but the large intrastudy variability in 24-hour total acid reflux may limit the usefulness of the method for assessment of therapeutic improvement.[22,50] However, Bennett et al.[4] showed that 1 g and 2 g of cimetidine, given for 12 weeks and compared with placebo, influenced significantly the number of reflux episodes, but not the other variables such as the mean duration of reflux episodes and the percentage of observations of pH >4.

Stomach

Gastric Secretion Measurement

Measurement of gastric secretion and the effect of drugs on acid output is a good example of the value of phase I dose finding studies in healthy volunteers to determine a target optimal therapeutic dose in patients in phase II and III therapeutic trials. The methods for gastric acid secretion analysis and meal-stimulated acid secretion, including quantitative 24-hour measurements, are well established, accurate and reproducible. In many clinical pharmacological studies the dose-dependent effect of drugs on pentagastrin-stimulated acid secretion in comparison with placebo has been demonstrated.[12] Under more physiological conditions, the effect of these compounds on food-stimulated acid secretion was shown.[36]

Long-Term Monitoring of Gastric pH (pH-Metry)

Prolonged measurements of gastric acidity are well suited for the evaluation of gastric antisecretory drugs. Until recently, this prolonged monitoring was done by intubation and aspiration. However, this required repeated sampling procedures which are inconvenient and uncomfortable for the subjects. Nocturnal sampling, especially when acid secretion is inhibited by drug intake, is often impossible as a result of low intragastric volumes.[28]

The recent development of stable, miniaturised glass electrodes and digital processing facilities has enabled the long-term reliable, safe and comfortable monitoring of intragastric pH in volunteers or patients.[14] The technique is very well suited for assessing the effect of antisecretory drugs on night secretion.

With this technique it was shown that a regimen of two doses of 300 mg of ranitidine did not lead to longer lasting inhibition of gastric pH than two doses of 150 mg.[46] This method provides precise pH-threshold 24-hour curves which give a precise indication of percentage of observations of pH >4 (considered necessary for ulcer healing) and so provides a more rational basis to compare the efficacy of different drugs.

Endoscopy (Ulcer Studies)

Endoscopy is an objective way of diagnosing peptic ulcer and its healing. However, the appreciation of the size of the ulcer can vary greatly from one investigator to another. This is why the only reliable endpoint for clinical efficacy is the complete disappearance of the ulcer with or without a scar.

It is important to realise that there is a strict correlation between ulcer healing rates and the potency of a drug to suppress acid secretion.[21] Better dose–response curves can be obtained when, additional to baseline and four-week endoscopies, an examination is performed also after two weeks. Few of the large double-blind trials in patients with peptic ulcer have been real dose finding studies. The reason for this is that investigators use strong antisecretory doses (based on pharmacodynamic dose finding studies) in the first trials and then progressively reduce the dosage in successive trials. For

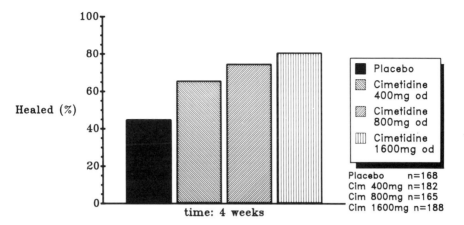

Figure 15.2. Dose-dependent effect of cimetidine on four-weeks' healing rates of duodenal ulcer. (Redrawn from data of Bravermann, 1986.[5])

example, 80 mg ranitidine decreases acid secretion by 70% in healthy volunteers, but the usual doses given to patients during clinical trials are 150 mg b.i.d. or 300 mg once daily (o.d.).

Concerning famotidine, a dose of 20 mg inhibits pentagastrin-stimulated secretion by 90%; this explains why Gitlen *et al.*[18] found no difference in the eight-week healing rate in patients with duodenal ulcers when comparing 20 mg b.i.d., 40 mg b.i.d. and 40 mg o.d. (82, 82 and 83% healing, respectively). In 1986, a large multicentre, double-blind placebo-controlled dose finding study was published which showed clearly that, in a total of 703 patients, cimetidine given once at bedtime accelerated duodenal ulcer healing in a dose-dependent manner after four weeks (*Figure 15.2*).[5] The design of the study was proposed by the Centre for Drug Evaluation and Research of the Food and Drug Administration.[41] This study is outstanding in numbers of patients and design, and has consequently led to the approval of the 800 mg single dose regimen (the 800 and 1600 mg doses were considered essentially indistinguishable).

Another study design was used to evaluate the efficacy of famotidine on the healing of duodenal ulcers in a total of 185 patients; in a double-blind randomised multicentre trial, 20 mg and 40 mg b.i.d., and 40 mg o.d. were compared with ranitidine 150 mg b.i.d. as reference drug. The healing after two weeks was 57%, 63%, 67% and 65%, respectively, and after four weeks was >80% in all groups. After eight weeks, healing was >90% in all groups and the results were not statistically different at any time.[35] With larger numbers of patients in the different treatment groups, statistically significant differences could possibly have become apparent.

Another placebo-controlled dose finding study compared different doses (35 µg b.i.d. and 70 µg b.i.d.) of enprostil at two and four weeks.[42] Recently a specific blocker of the enzyme $H^+ K^+$-ATP-ase (the gastric proton pump) in the parietal cell, omeprazole, has been introduced in the therapy of peptic ulcer. This substance binds strongly for periods longer than 16 hours and this explains why the antisecretory effect persists a long time after the substance has disappeared from the blood stream. Moreover, its antisecretory activity increases after a few days because omeprazole increases its own availability by inhibiting acid secretion.[30]

These interesting characteristics explain why the antisecretory effect of omeprazole does not correlate with C_{max}, but with AUC in a non-linear fashion.[33] In a carefully designed dose finding study of 43 patients with duodenal ulcer, the administration of 20, 30, 40 or 60 mg/day induced healing in >90% in the four groups.[6] This absence of dose effect can be explained by the already strong inhibitory effect of 20 mg (more than 90% in volunteers). However, a linear correlation between the dose and response is observed between doses (10–60 mg/day) after two weeks of treatment (healing rates between 50 and 100%). The first dose finding study in acute gastric ulcer healing was carried out using omeprazole 20 mg and 40 mg *nocti*, respectively, compared with ranitidine 2 × 150 mg.[45] Omeprazole turned out to be superior at both doses.

Antacid treatment and its dose–response relationship was analysed in a well-designed study as recently as 1984.[26] A group of 107 patients with acute duodenal ulcer received 7.5, 15 or 30 ml of a liquid aluminium/magnesium hydroxide or placebo six times a day. After four weeks, only 29% of the patients had a healed ulcer on placebo, while healing rates with antacid were 46(n.s.), 85% and 88% (p <0.001), respectively. Drug-related side effects were recorded only in the group with the highest dose regimen. Thus, an optimum antacid requirement of 90 ml per day was identified for the treatment of duodenal ulcer (acid neutralising capacity 207 mmol HCl).

Dose Finding Studies in Prevention of Recurrence of Peptic Ulcer

The first large dose-finding study of prevention of duodenal ulcer was published in 1984 by Sontag and others.[38] In a double-blind randomised placebo-controlled multicentre trial, cimetidine 200 mg and 300 mg b.i.d. and a different dose regimen (400 mg o.d.) were compared with placebo in 370 patients. By the end of one year, the cumulative symptomatic recurrence rate (demonstrated by endoscopy) was similar for all three doses (19%, 15% and 13%, respectively), while under placebo the recurrence rate was 34.7% (p <0.01).

Endoscopy (NSAID-lesion prevention studies)

Endoscopy is the most accurate way to analyse the therapeutic and preventive effect of protective substances on lesions induced by non-steroidal anti-inflammatory drugs (NSAIDs). This model has been validated by several authors, although different scores of lesions have been used.[27,34]

Several new prostaglandins have been tested prophylactically or therapeutically against the gastric lesions induced by acetylsalicylic acid (ASA). Gilbert *et al.*[16] showed a clear dose response between the dose of prostaglandin PGE_2 and the proportion of volunteers with minimal or no gastroduodenal lesion induced by 1.3 g of ASA. By endoscopic examination, using a toxicity score, a clear therapeutic (preventive) dose response was described.[43]

Gastric Potential Difference (GPD)

Measurement of the gastric transmucosal potential difference is an easy and well-tolerated technique. The GPD is a very sensitive index of mucosal integrity.

A good correlation between the kinetics of the ASA-induced drop of GPD and the percentage of damaged cells shown with light microscopy has been demonstrated in healthy volunteers by Baskin and others.[1] In volunteers, we have used this technique to show a dose-dependent reduction of the area under the curve (AUC) of the GPD by two doses of rioprostil, and a reduction of the drop in GPD following the ingestion of 0.5 g of ASA given with rioprostil.[11] Vance and others[44] have demonstrated a linear correlation between the bioavailability of ASA and the AUC of GPD.

Faecal Occult Blood-Loss Measurement (^{51}Cr-Labelled Red Blood Cells)

The quantitative measurement of ^{51}Cr activity in the stool after i.v. administration of ^{51}Cr-labelled red blood cells as a measure of faecal occult blood-loss in man is a sensitive and internationally well-established and accepted method. As an example, a dose-dependent protective effect of the PGE_1-analogue rioprostil on occult blood loss after high doses of ASA has been shown.[9]

Methods for Analysing Gastric Emptying

Several methods can be used to study this parameter (*Table 15.1*). The scintigraphic isotopic method is the 'gold standard'. Its principle lies in the detection by a gamma camera of photons emitted by one or two radioactive isotopes which have been incorporated into the solid and liquid phases of a meal. Practically, digestible solids are marked *in vitro* with ^{99}technetium, the liquids by indium DTPA and the lipids can also be marked by ^{75}selemium. With the help of a computer, the emptying slopes or the half-time of emptying of each specific isotope can be calculated. This method is non-invasive and sensitive. However, it is expensive and difficult to perform.

In a recent study, Santander *et al.*[31] compared the sensitivity of measurement of gastric emptying of liquids and solids by isotopic techniques, and of gastrointestinal motility by manometric methods, assessing the effect of nifedipine, 30 mg, versus placebo on these parameters. No effect was observed on gastric emptying measurement while manometry demonstrated that antral motility was significantly inhibited and duodenal motility increased. The authors concluded that either gastroduodenal changes are not severe enough to alter emptying or isotopic techniques are not sensitive enough to detect subtle changes in gastric emptying.

According to Fisher and Malmud[15], scintigraphic emptying tests are useful to explore the effects of various drugs. Three other methods are available for measuring gastric emptying: radiopaque markers, gastric impedance and sonography. However, these techniques are not yet validated and their precise sensitivity to modification by drugs is not known.

Table 15.1. Methods of measurement of gastric emptying (GE).

Techniques	Advantage(s)	Limitation(s)
1. Intubation and perfusion of markers (PSP, PEG, Isotopes)	Measurement of gastric secretion, emptying and intestinal absorption	Analysis only GE of liquids Invasive
2. Double isotope technique (isotopic scintiscan;[99] Tc for solids,[111] Ind for liquids,[75] Se for lipids)	Very precise Analysis of GE + intestinal absorption Analysis of both liquid and solid emptying Non-invasive	Limited to research Expensive Difficult
3. Radiopaque marker	Simple Reproducible Non-expensive	Interdigestion period Not yet validated
4. Gastic impedance		Not yet validated
5. Sonography: post-prandial measurement of astric surface	Simple Non-invasive	Not yet validated

Older methods, like gastroduodenal intubation with the slow perfusion of several markers, are very precise and permit the simultaneous measurement of gastric secretion, gastric emptying and intestinal absorption. However, they are invasive, unpleasant and limited to specific research questions.

Biliary Tract

Gallbladder Sonography

For the evaluation of drug effects on gallbladder motility, sonography is used. The total plane of the gallbladder and its changes after drug administration are measured by planimetry. According to Hopman et al.[20], serial sonography is an easily performed, reliable and sensitive method by which to measure gallbladder contraction without the disadvantage of radiation or intubation. They showed a direct correlation between increasing physiological doses of cholecystokinin (CCK) and gallbladder emptying. The time-consuming calculation required to measure the gallbladder volumes can be reduced by using a computerised technique to calculate the sum of cylinders.[19]

This technique has also been used to analyse the relaxing effect of the calcium antagonist nifedipine on the contractile effect induced by CCK.[29]

Sphincter of Oddi Endoscopic Manometry

Endoscopic manometry permits direct recording and quantification of the sphincter of Oddi motility after the administration of drugs. It is an invasive procedure which has been used to test the effect of modern analgesic drugs (like tramadol, pentazocine and buprenorphine) on the bile duct sphincter motor activity.[40] In this study it was shown that pentazocine increased significantly the sphincter pressure and was contraindicated during ERCP.

Small Bowel

Several techniques are now available to measure the transit time (*Table 15.2*).

H_2-breath test is an easy and useful method to measure the mouth-to-caecum transit time in volunteers or patients. However, its variability is high and is probably not reproducible enough to be used as a tool for pharmacological dose–response studies (it could be used as a screening test). To our knowledge, no dose finding studies have yet been published using this method.

The scintigraphic determination of the small intestinal transit time with lactulose containing ^{99}technetium DTPA allows a more accurate determination of the gastrocaecal time than the H_2-breath technique.[7] It has the advantage that it can quantify gastric emptying and the small intestinal transit

Table 15.2. Techniques for studying small and large bowel transit time.

A. *Breath tests*

	Site of entry	Measurement	Analytical method
1. Lactulose	Colon	H_2, Breath	Gas chromatograph
2. Xylose	Duodenum	Xylose, Blood	Colorimetry

Difference between 1 and 2 equals the small intestinal transit

Advantages:
  Easy, inexpensive, no radioactivity
Limitations:
  Problem of non H_2-producers: up to 25%
  Interference by diet, antibiotics
  Only liquid meals
  May lack the desired sensitivity for pharmacological studies
  Cannot determine precisely the importance of gastric emptying in the total
    gastrocolic time

B. *Scintigraphy*

Lactulose with ^{99m} Technetium

Advantages with breath technique:
  Determination of gastric emptying *and* small intestinal transit time
  Accurate
  Sensitive (needs confirmation)
Disadvantages:
  Large amount of radioactivity
  Interpretations sometimes difficult (overlapping)

time. The combination with the determination of gastric emptying is useful, as the authors showed that the individual variations in small intestinal transit time were correlated with individual variations in gastric emptying.

Large Bowel (Endoscopy)

Recently, a well-designed double-blind, placebo-controlled therapeutic dose–response study was carried out in a total of 87 patients with mild to moderate active ulcerative colitis.[32] In comparison with placebo, 1.6 g and 4.8 g of 5-aminosalicylic acid (5-ASA) increased complete and partial healing of chronic ulcerative colitis dose-dependently (*Figure 15.3*).

Maintenance treatment and its dose–response relationship were analysed by Khan *et al.* in 1980[24], when 170 patients with ulcerative colitis were allotted at random to treatment groups of 1.2 or 4 g sulphasalazine daily (no placebo group). The optimum therapeutic dose to maintain remission turned out to be 2 g daily as the relapse rate after six months by clinical, endoscopical and histological assessment was significantly lower (14%) than with 1 g/day (34%). With 4 g/day, results were improved further (9%), but at the expense of frequent side-effects.

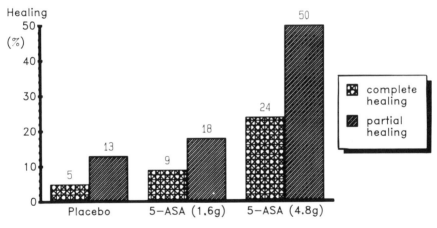

Figure 15.3. Effect of oral 5-aminosalicylic acid (5-ASA) therapy on mildly to moderately active ulcerative colitis. (Redrawn from data of Schröder *et al.*, 1987.[32])

Conclusion

Therapeutic dose finding studies to determine the optimal dosage regimen for the treatment of gastrointestinal diseases have been carried out only in the past few years. Previously, large numbers of clinical studies had been performed (e.g. in peptic ulcer disease), comparing one dose of an investigational drug with placebo and/or one dose of a standard drug, without addressing the rationale for dosage and/or dosage regimens. It is obvious that the recent change of approach to the therapeutic evaluation of a new drug reflects also a strong impact of the requirements of the health authorities in different countries.

Various methods in clinical pharmacology which have a high predictability make a first estimate of therapeutic doses possible and should be used for the development of new drugs and new indications for known compounds. Nevertheless, therapeutic dose finding studies for validation of the therapeutic dose and determination of optimal dosage regimen are ultimately necessary. Adequate and well-designed dose–response studies have a strong impact on the therapeutic decision. Therefore, for scientific as well as for ethical reasons, more trials of this kind are needed.

Acknowledgements

We are indebted to Mr B. Frankenberger for technical assistance and Mrs M. Berner for typing the manuscript.

References

[1] Baskin, W. N., Ivey, K.J., Krause, W.J., Jeffrey, G.E., and Gemmell, R.T. Aspirin-induced ultrastructural changes in human gastric mucosa. Correlation with potential difference. *Ann. Int. Med.*, **85**, 299–303, 1976.

[2] Baunack, A.R., Demol, P., and Weihrauch, T.R., Placebo-controlled comparison of the efficacy of the calcium antagonists Bay 1 8201 and nifedipine on the lower esophageal sphincter pressure (LESP) in volunteers. *Gastroenterology*, **88**, 1319, 1985.

[3] Baunack, A.R., Froese, G., Demol, P., Wargenau, M., Ruoff, H.J., and Weihrauch, T.R. Effect of rioprostil, an oral prostaglandin E1 (PGE1) analogue, on lower esophageal sphincter pressure and on the motility of the distal esophagus in healthy volunteers. *Z. Gastroent.*, **26**, 199–203, 1988.

[4] Bennett, J.R., Buckton, G., and Martin, H.D. Cimetidine in gastro-oesophageal reflux. *Digestion*, **26**, 166–72, 1983.

[5] Braverman, A.J. Dose validation and study design criteria in current cimetidine studies. *Clin. Ther.*, **8** (Suppl. A), 49–56, 1986.

[6] British Cooperative Study. Omeprazole in duodenal ulceration: acid inhibition, symptom relief, endoscopic healing and recurrence. *Brit. Med. J.*, **289**, 525–8, 1984.

[7] Caride, V.J., Prokop, E.K., Troncale, F.J., Buddoura, W., Winchenbach, K., and McCallum, R.W. Scintigraphic determination of small intestinal transit time: comparison with the hydrogen breath technique. *Gastroenterology*, **86**, 714–20, 1984.

[8] Castell, D.O., Richter, J.E., and Boag Dalton, C. *Esophageal Motility Testing*. Elsevier, New York, Amsterdam, London, 35–78, 1987.

[9] Cohen, A., Salzmann, P.M., Brady, C.L., Simon, D.M., and McCormack, G.H. Effect of rioprostil on aspirin-induced gastrointestinal blood loss in normal volunteers. *J. Clin. Pharmacol*, **24**, 401, 1984.

[10] Cohen, S., Morris, D.W., Schoen, H.J., and DiMarino, A.J. The effect of oral and intravenous metoclopramide on human lower oesophageal sphincter pressure. *Gastroenterology*, **70**, 484–7, 1976.

[11] Demol, P., Schmitz, H.D., Weihrauch, T.R., and Kuhlmann, J. Prevention of the acetylsalicylic acid-induced changes of the gastric potential difference by the new synthetic prostaglandin E1 analogue rioprostil. *Arzneim-Forsch/Drug Res.*, **36**, 1406–8, 1986.

[12] Demol, P., Wingender, W., Weihrauch, T.R., and Graefe, K.H. Inhibition of gastric secretion in man by rioprostil, a new synthetic methyl prostaglandin E1. *Arzneim-Forsch/Drug Res.*, **35**, 839–43, 1985.

[13] FDA Guideline. *Guideline for the Format and Content of the Clinical and Statistical Sections of New Drug Applications.* Center for Drug Evaluation and Research, Food and Drug Administration, Department of Health and Human Services, 15, 1988.

[14] Fimmel, C.J., Etienne, A., Cilluffo, T., von Ritter, C., Gasser, T., Rey, J.P., Caradonna-Moscatelli, P., Sabbatini, F., Pace, F., Bühler, H.W., Bauerfeind, P., and Blum, A.L. Long-term ambulatory gastric pH monitoring: validation of a new method and effect of H2-antagonists. *Gastroenterology*, **88**, 1842–51, 1985.

[15] Fisher, R.S. and Malmud, L.S. Scintigraphic techniques for the study of gastrointestinal motor function. *Adv. Int. Med.*, **31**, 395–418, 1986.

[16] Gilbert, D.A., Surawicz, G.M., Silverstein, F.E., Weinberg, C.R., Saunders, D.R., Feld, A.D., Sanford, R.L., Bergman, D., and Washington, P. Prevention of acute aspirin-induced gastric mucosal injury by 15-R-15 methyl prostaglandin E2: an endoscopic study. *Gastroenterology*, **86**, 339–45, 1984.

[17] Gilbert, R.J., Dodds, W.J., Kahrilas, P.J., Hogan, W.J., and Lipman, S. Effect of cisapride, a new prokinetic agent, on esophageal motor function. *Dig. Dis. Sci.*, **32**, 1331–6, 1987.

[18] Gitlin, N., Mucullough, A.J., and Smith, J.L. Multiclinic double-blind dose ranging study evaluating the efficacy and safety of famotidine in the healing of active duodenal ulcer as compared to placebo. *Americ. J. Gastroent.*, **80**, 840, 1985.

[19] Hopman, W.P.M., Brouwer, W.F.M., Rosenbusch, G., Jansen, J.B.M.J., and Lamers, C.B.H.W. A computerised method for rapid quantification of gallbladder volume from real-time sonographs. *Radiology*, **154**, 236–7, 1985.

[20] Hopman, W.P.M., Kerstens, P.J.S.M., Jansen, J.B.M.J., Rosenbusch, G., and Lamers, C.B.H.W. Effect of graded physiologic doses of cholecystokinin on gallbladder contraction measured by ultrasonography. *Gastroenterology*, **89**, 1242–7, 1985.

[21] Hunt, R.H., Howden, C.W., Jones, D.B., Burget, D.W., and Kerr, G.D. The correlation between acid suppression and peptic ulcer healing. *Scand. J. Gastroent.*, **12** (Suppl. 125), 22–31, 1987.

[22] Johnsson, F. and Joelsson, B. Reproducibility of ambulatory oesophageal pH monitoring. *GUT*, **29**, 886–9, 1988.

[23] Kaul, B., Petersen, H., Erichsen, H., Myrvold, H.E., Grette, K., Halvorsen, T., and Fjosne, U. Gastro-oesophageal reflux disease. *Scand. J. Gastroent.*, **21**, 139–45, 1986.

[24] Khan, A.K.A., Howes, D.T., Piris, J., and Truelove, S.C. Optimum dose of sulphasalazine for maintenance treatment in ulcerative colitis. *GUT*, **21**, 232–40, 1980.

[25] Kilbinger, H. and Weilhrauch, T.R. Drugs increasing gastrointestinal motility. *Pharmacology*, **25**, 61–72, 1982.

[26] Kumar, N., Vij, J.C., Karol, A., and Anand, B.S. Controlled therapeutic

trial to determine the optimum dose of antacids in duodenal ulcer. *GUT*, **25**, 1199–1202, 1984.

[27] Lanza, F.L., Royer, G.L., and Nelson, B.S. Endoscopic evaluation of the effects of aspirin, buffered aspirin and enteric-coated aspirin on gastric duodenal mucosa. *New Eng. J. Med.*, **303**, 136–8, 1980.

[28] Levin, E., Kirsner, J.B., Palmer, W.L., and Butler, C. The variability and periodicity of the nocturnal gastric secretion in normal individuals. *Gastroenterology*, **10**, 939–51, 1948.

[29] Porshen, R., Pieper, S., Bernhardt, L., Schade, B., and Wienbeck, M. *In vivo* effects of nifedipine and BAY i 8201 on caerulein induced gallbladder contraction. *Z. Gastroent.*, **26**, 755–61, 1988.

[30] Prichard, P.J., Yeomans, N.D., Mihaly, G.W., Jones, D.B., Buckle, P.J., Smallwood, R.A., and Louis, W.J. Omeprazole: a study of its inhibition of gastric pH and oral pharmacokinetics after morning or evening dosage. *Gastroenterology*, **88**, 64–9, 1985.

[31] Santander, R., Mena, I., Gramisu, M., and Valenzuela, J.E. Effect of nifedipine on gastric emptying and gastrointestinal motility in man. *Dig. Dis. Sci*, **33**, 535–9, 1988.

[32] Schröder, K.W., Tremaine, W.J., and Ilstrup, D.M. Coated oral 5-aminosalicylic acid therapy for mildly to moderately active ulcerative colitis. *New Eng. J. Med.*, **317**, 1625–9, 1987.

[33] Sharma, B.K., Walt, R.P., Pounder, R.E., Gomes, M. de F., Wood, E.C., and Logan, E.H. Optimal dose of oral omeprazole for maximal 24-hour decrease of intragastric acidity. *GUT*, **25**, 957–64, 1984.

[34] Silverstein, F.E., Gilbert, D.A., Surawicz, C.S., Ring, C.E., Feld, A.D., Sanford, R.L., and Saunders, D.R. Prostaglandin E2 (PGE2) cytoprotection in aspirin-induced gastric mucosal injury: an endoscopic study. *Am. J. Gastroent*, **74**, 93, 1980.

[35] Simon, B., Dammann, H.G., Jakob, G., Miederer, S.E. *et al.* Famotidin versus Ranitidin in der Akutbehandlung der Ulcus-duodeni-Erkrankung. Eine Multizenter-Vergleichsstudie in Deutschland. *Z. Gastroent.*, **23**, 47–51, 1985.

[36] Singer, M.V., Schulte, H., Demol, P., Eysselein, V., and Goebell, H. Dose–response effects of rioprostil, a new synthetic methyl prostaglandin E1 on gastric acid secretion and release of gastrin in humans. *Gastroenterology*, **88**, 1588, 1985.

[37] Smart, H.L., James, P.D., Atkinson, M., and Hawkey, C.J. Treatment of reflux eosophagitis with a prostaglandin analogue. *GUT*, **28**, 1358–9, 1987.

[38] Sontag, S., Graham, D.Y., Belsito, A., *et al.* Cimetidine, cigarette smoking, and recurrence of duodenal ulcer. *New Eng. J. Med.*, **311**, 689–93, 1984.

[39] Stanciu, C. and Bennett, J.R. Metoclopramide in gastro-oesophageal reflux. *GUT*, **14**, 275–79, 1973.

[40] Staritz, M., Poralla, T., Manns, M., and Meyer zum Buschenfelde, K.H. Effect of modern analgesic drugs (tramadol, pentazocine and buprenorphine) on the bile duct sphincter in man. *GUT*, **27**, 567–9, 1986.

[41] Temple, R. Personal communication. Office of Drug Evaluation I, Center for Drug Evaluation and Research, Food and Drug Administration, USA, 1988.

[42] Thomson, A.B.R. Treatment of duodenal ulcer with enprostil, a synthetic prostaglandin E2 analogue. *Am. J. Med.* **81**, 59–63, 1986.

[43] Tolman, K.G., Detweiler, M.K., Harrison, C.A., Rollins, D.E., Simon, D.A., Brady, C., McCormack, G.H., and Bryant, E.C. Effect of rioprostil on aspirin-induced gastrointestinal mucosal changes in normal volunteers. *J. Clin. Pharmacol.*, **28**, 76–80, 1988.

[44] Vance, J., Luecker, P.W., Tilling, W., Procaccini, R., and Wetzelsberger, N. The transmural gastric potential difference in combination with pharmacokinetic profiles. A new approach to combine kinetic and dynamic properties of compounds. *Meth. Find. Exp. Cl. Ph.*, **4**, 533–8, 1982.

[45] Walan, A., Bader, J.P., Classen, M., Lamers, C.B.H.W., Piper, D.W., Rutgersson, K., and Eriksson, S. Effect of omeprazole and ranitidine on ulcer healing and relapse rates in patients with benign gastric ulcer. *New Engl. J. Med.*, **320**, 69–75, 1989.

[46] Walt, R.P., Male, P.J., Rawlings, J., Hunt, R.H., Milton-Thompson, G.J., and Misiewicz, J.J. Comparison of the effects of ranitidine, cimetidine and placebo on the 24-hour intragastric acidity and nocturnal acid secretion in patients with duodenal ulcer. *GUT*, **22**, 49–54, 1981.

[47] Weihrauch, T.R. Esophageal manometry. In *Encyclopedia of Medical Devices and Instrumentation*, J.G. Webster (ed), Wiley & Sons, New York, 1236–45, 1988.

[48] Weihrauch, T.R. and Demol, P. Pharmacological dose–response curves in gastrointestinal therapy. *Dose–response Relationships in Man*, Esteve Foundation Symposium III, Son Vida/Mallorca, 1988.

[49] Weihrauch, T.R., Förster, C.F., and Krieglstein, J. Evaluation of the effect of domperidone on human oesophageal and gastroduodenal motility by intraluminal manometry. *Postgrad. Med. J.*, **55** (Suppl. 1), 7–10, 1979.

[50] Wiener, G.J., Morgan, T.M., Copper, J.B. *et al.*. Ambulatory 24-hour esophageal pH monitoring. Reproducibility and variability of pH parameters. *Dig. Dis. Sci.*, **33**, 1127–33, 1988.

16. The Importance of Pharmacodynamic Studies in Phase I Trials

R. F. Drucker

In phase I drug trials, emphasis is placed typically on the assessment of human tolerance, as well as on the absorption, distribution, metabolism and excretion of drugs. I believe that this is because of the widespread perception that presently available methods of measuring drug response lack the necessary sensitivity or therapeutic relevance, and that extrapolation from a volunteer subject to a patient population is somehow inappropriate. This has often resulted in phases I and II not being planned as a continuum, and has added to the pharmaceutical industry's reluctance to develop or use 'surrogate' clinical endpoints. However, substantial technological and methodological advances have resulted in renewed emphasis on human pharmacodynamic studies, and have enabled phase I testing to become more effective and efficient. Apart from the obvious economies of time, this has obviated the need to expose large numbers of patients unnecessarily to a drug that may have fundamental flaws.

I will attempt to highlight the increased importance of phase I pharmacodynamic trials, using pertinent examples drawn from the published literature, in particular, from recent issues of the *British Journal of Clinical Pharmacology*. Many of these examples are based on the use of so-called 'surrogate' end-points. This is where the investigator has reason to believe that a particular response, perhaps a laboratory measurement in the healthy volunteer, correlates in some way with the desired therapeutic response. One example would be where the leukotrienes have been implicated in a particular disease state, and a putative leukotriene synthesis inhibitor is to be tested. Under such circumstances, it is not unreasonable to think that, if inhibition of leukotriene synthesis can be demonstrated in normal subjects, the drug may indeed have a clinical effect in patients. Of course, this does not address the larger issue, namely, that when a drug is studied in patients one is almost always dealing with multifactor disease states.

Just as primary pharmacology relates to the desired therapeutic response, general pharmacological properties (i.e., secondary pharmacology) of the drug may provide a pointer to other therapeutic utilities. Although such properties may also impinge on the issue of associated risk, it is very difficult to obtain valid information on safety in phase I. In addition, a number of important issues depend upon balance and judgement. For example, with all the non-invasive techniques available currently for assessing a variety of body functions, in true futuristic fashion we could measure everything on everybody, everytime we give a drug in phase I.

Clearly, there is no substitute for thought, but crudely, in terms of general pharmacology, what we really want to know is the nature and magnitude of the effect on critical body systems – whether an important response is occurring in the cardiovascular system, for instance. Does the drug do anything specifically to the heart rate or stroke volume and thereby affect cardiac output, for example, or does it do anything to peripheral resistance? These are important observations with respect to the cardiovascular system. Also, will the respiratory system be affected? Does the drug have any effect on rate and depth of respiration and, perhaps more importantly, respiratory drive?

My particular biases are that you cannot do everything in one study, that you do not want to generate shaky information on which to base decision-making. This is to say, that any particular study will clearly have a given degree of sensitivity and specificity with regard to a question, and this can almost always be identified prospectively; sensitivity and specificity of the study should be such that the question posed can be addressed and intelligent decisions can be based upon the results. In the real world of phase I investigation, such studies are undertaken because they produce results that relate to what may be identified as a positive, negative or an equivocal outcome. You should be able to identify, a priori, what will be positive or negative. If you cannot, the study should be stopped. Phase I is not a field for self-indulgent dilettantes or for those interested only in the academic satisfaction of taking a novel entity into man for the first time.

I would now like to cite selected pharmacodynamic approaches to exemplify the points I have been making, and would emphasise that merely obtaining the observation is only part of the job. Not only must the data be analysed in isolation as it relates to a given variable, but we must also look across different and seemingly unrelated variables for patterns of pharmacodynamic response. With the advent of the 'neurocomputer', we now have technology to do just this, the element of time previously having made it prohibitive. The point is that we must elevate the status of observations obtained from pharmacodynamic studies to the realm of information. For example, the neurocomputer can identify the fact that there is a repetitive pattern in a given percentage of volunteers who develop increased blood pressure after dosing, and two days after completion of the study show increased liver function tests (LFTs), though both could remain within normal range. I can speculate why increased blood pressure and increased LFTs within normal range might occur, but it is not an association that I would usually look for. Neurocomputer systems mimic the ability of the human brain to learn from experience, and can highlight such an association. They excel at recognising subtle, hard-to-define patterns and, as such, these observations should be taken seriously.

While the equipment needed for nuclear magnetic resonance (NMR) studies is expensive, the type and quality of information obtained can provide much new data for the clinical pharmacologist. Apart from static morphological uses, that is diagnosis, the technique is of great utility to the clinical pharmacologist in the assessment of cardiovascular changes. These dynamic images can reflect alterations in cardiac cycle and blood flow, and information is available on stroke volume, ejection fraction, ventricular filling and ejection rates. This is made possible by the fact that high quality, reproducible images can be obtained repeatedly over prolonged study periods. Aellig[2] has suggested that this technology represents possibly the most accurate method for the non-invasive assessment of ventricular volumes, and for the determination of ventricular mass.

Aellig[2] also predicted that NMR spectroscopy will prove very useful in determining dynamic changes in the chemical composition of organs, such as the heart and brain. Use of ^{31}P-MRS to measure (in vivo) high energy phosphate metabolism in the human heart, provides a non-invasive method for the assessment of cellular energy reserve in myocardial infarction, and thereby can measure metabolic response to drug intervention. The neurological counterpart of this would be the assessment of treatment for acute cerebral ischaemia. With time and improvements in technology, it is expected that drug concentrations in the various organs of the human body will be measured directly with NMR spectroscopy.

The effects of an i.v. infusion of adrenaline and of mental stress evoked by a colour word test were investigated in healthy volunteers by Larsson et al.[7] Mental stress was evoked by a modified video-taped version of Stroop's colour word conflict test. Blood sampling and blood pressure measurements were then performed at 5 min intervals. As expected, high physiological levels of circulating adrenaline, but not mental stress, elicited biphasic changes in functional response to β-adrenoceptor stimulation in lymphocytes, and no changes in antagonism or agonist binding in platelet adrenoceptors. It has been suggested that such techniques might be used to differentiate between the tissue selectivity of various types of drugs that act on the β-adrenoceptor system.

It has been found that Doppler wave form analysis can provide a simple and reproducible method for studying indices related to blood flow. While it is theoretically possible to calculate volume flow directly, if the diameter of a vessel is known, this measure has been found to be too inaccurate to provide reproducible measurements. Usually, the pulsatility index (PI) and maximum (centre stream) velocity are measured. In the case of measurements from the renal artery, the vessel is first visualised by real-time scanning, in contrast to other vessels which can be identified anatomically. In a study reported by MacDonald et al.[9], regional blood velocity was measured in the common and internal carotid, femoral and renal arteries. Blood pressure and heart rate were recorded with a semi-automated sphygmomanometer, and blood velocity indices were determined with an ultrasound scanner. The latter permitted the selective effects of human alpha calcitonin gene-related peptide to be documented.

In elderly patients, cumulative doses of inhaled salbutamol have been reported by Lipworth et al.[8] to result in a dose-dependent increase in finger tremor as well as in heart rate, along with a fall in plasma potassium. This study demonstrated that there was no evidence of decreased sensitivity of the beta-2 adrenoceptor response in elderly patients. Accordingly, the approach can also be used to measure and extrapolate from the activity of similar types of drugs in healthy young volunteers.

Measuring the onset of action of nitrates has always been a problem and antianginal potency correlates poorly with plasma nitroglycerin concentrations. Better measurements can now be made using a microcomputer-based heart rate transmitter device and receiver, as described by Lahtela & Sotaniemi[6], who measured heart rate transdermally from the precordial region. The microcomputer technology used proved to be reliable, simple and relatively inexpensive, and clearly has wider application in phase I clinical studies.

The pharmacodynamic properties of psychopharmacological agents can be investigated in phase I studies. Thus, Wildin et al.[13] used ventilatory response to CO_2 inhalation and psychomotor performance tests as pharmacodynamic indices of the effect of new benzodiazepines. In conjunction with more standard observations on pulse, blood pressure and body temperature, respiratory changes were measured by analysis of the ventilation curve. Pharmacodynamic actions were related to plasma concentrations of the drugs. Psychomotor performance was also measured in the same study using a number of quantitative test systems. These included a measure of the reaction time required by a subject to scan a semicircle of six lights adjacent to corresponding buttons. Lights were illuminated individually and, on a random basis, the subject was expected to release the baseline button and to press the appropriate response button in order to extinguish the light. In this way, both recognition time and response time were measured separately. More classic tests included the digit symbol substitution test (Wechsler), involving the substitution of symbols for digits according to a prescribed code. In addition, the subjects reported their subjective condition on visual analogue scales. A measure of postural stability or sway was also included. In this way, psychopharmacological agents were characterised according to 'surrogate' pharmacodynamic effects in addition to the usual psychological profiling.

A subjective 'minor symptom evaluation' (MSE) profile has been used to detect subtle changes in symptoms subsequent to dosing with beta-blockers. It was concluded from studies by Dimenas et al.[4] that there was no difference between atenolol and metoprolol with respect to mild subjective symptoms, but that duration of pharmacodynamic effects did seem to be consistent with relative elimination half-lives. The clinical implication of this study is that high plasma drug concentrations should be avoided and the drugs should not be given at night or late in the evening.

Information relating to the effects of drugs on the gastrointestinal tract tends not to be fully appreciated. Recognising that a selective receptor antagonist of 5-hydroxytryptamine can be shown to exert marked gastrointestinal motility effects in animals, colonic pressures were recorded in normal volunteers by Stacher et al.[12] They used a disposable multilumen catheter assembly, with constant distilled water perfusion from a capillary hydraulic infusion system. Sudden occlusion of the perfusion catheters produced a pressure rise that could be recorded with conventional transducers. Analysis was then performed using a computer program that determined the mean capillary baseline pressure, the number, mean amplitude and mean duration of contractions, as well as the area under the pressure curve for each test period. Respiration was monitored using a Beckman strain gauge pneumograph, and respiratory artifacts were eliminated by visual inspection. In this way, significant drug effects on the motor activity of the human sigmoid colon were measured.

A variety of drugs are known to influence gastric emptying. For instance, post-operative use of opioids is a serious cause of delayed emptying, and the development of compounds that can diminish these effects could be of particular interest. In addition, a number of hormones that affect gastrointestinal motility are believed to be of considerable importance, and will be a possible source of future drugs. Petring[10] measured gastric emptying in normal volunteers following an overnight fast, in a study where the subjects were given a semi-solid meal labelled with Tc-99m resin. Motility or emptying was then studied in the anterior projection using a gamma camera with a low energy, parallel-hole collimator. A succession of images was obtained over a 90 min period.

A relatively simple system for measuring gastric mucosal damage commonly associated with the use of low doses of aspirin and non-steroidal anti-inflammatory agents has been described by Kitchingman et al.[5] Gastric injury was measured as the rate of mucosal bleeding over time using a relatively simple gastric washing technique. Phenol red was introduced into the stomach at each sampling period to act as a recovery marker. The dye was assayed spectrophotometrically and the washings were assayed for haemoglobin. The proportion of phenol red recovered in the washes was then used to adjust haemoglobin assays for antegrade loss through the pylorus or for failure in aspiration. Such techniques are particularly relevant to assessing agents with gastric irritant potential which may be used in the treatment of rheumatoid arthritis or for prophylaxis against myocardial or cerebral infarction.

Surrogate endpoints for the effects of drugs on the endocrine system are well established. There is currently much interest in novel dopamine D2-receptor agonists. As dopamine receptors are located, among other places, on the lactotrophs of the anterior pituitary, and dopamine plays a role in the inhibition of prolactin release, serum prolactin levels may be used as an indicator of activity. In a study reported by Acton and Broom[1], relatively small doses of a D2-receptor agonist produced a statistically significant lowering of both basal and food-stimulated serum prolactin levels relative to placebo in healthy volunteers. Al-Sereiti et al.[3] have shown that topical bromocriptine, a dopamine-2 receptor agonist, can effectively lower intraocular pressure in normal eyes as measured by non-contact tonometry, and that this could represent a relatively simple method for measuring the activity of this class of drugs.

Histamine is a known regulator of the immune response following antigenic stimulation. In delayed hypersensitivity reactions, this is caused partly by stimulation of the histamine H_2-receptors on T-suppressor and cytolytic-T cells. A histamine H_2-receptor antagonist, e.g. cimetidine, can inhibit the immune suppression mediated by T cells. The challenge is to verify the immune-enhancing effect of cimetidine in healthy individuals and to correlate, in vivo, the time sequence of antigenic stimulation to the immune modulatory effect using a recognised cell-mediated immune reaction – namely the tuberculin skin test. Synman et al.[11] have shown that it is possible for a histamine H_2-receptor blocker to modulate T-suppressor cell function selectively. A regimen of cimetidine, administered in advance of antigenic stimulation, was reported to enhance the delayed-type hypersensitivity reaction in healthy volunteers.

Having made reference to a range of techniques relating to primary and secondary pharmacology, I would like to go on record as saying that I do not believe that all of these or other techniques can or should be included in phase I studies, or that all or any should necessarily be applied to any particular drug. It is a fallacy that undertaking the minimum number of studies, and trying to measure everything on everybody, affords the most efficient way to develop drugs. There is no substitute for thought; no substitute for studies based on specific questions. The idea that one comprehensive study, where everything is measured and all of the numbers are input into a computer, will somehow come up with the appropriate answers is naive. What we must do is develop coherent phase I trial programmes, responsive to the available preclinical data and projected therapeutic utility.

The major test of everything I have said about phase I pharmacodynamic studies is the extent to which they are responsive to the following issues:

• While information on safety derived from phase I studies may be limited, establishment of a phase I pharmacological (pharmacodynamic) profile provides a more rational basis for dosage form and dosage regimen selection in phase II.
• The pharmacodynamic profile can also supply information relative to the appropriateness of the clinical indications to be studied and the comparators chosen for phase II.
• Particular features of the drug observed in phase I can be focused on in phase II studies.

In conclusion, there is no substitute for careful thought in applying pharmacodynamic measurements in phase I clinical research. I am totally opposed to any suggestion that there is a pharmacodynamic test battery that can be mindlessly applied in all instances. Whenever confronted with the goal of planning a phase I prgramme, including pharmacodynamic studies, we should always ask 'What do we need to know about the human pharmacology of this drug, may this information be generated appropriately during phase I, and, if so, how?' The phase I programme and its components should always be considered in the context of the total drug development process.

References

[1] Acton, G. and Broom, C. A dose rising study of the safety and effects on serum prolactin of SK&F 101468, a novel dopamine D_2-receptor agonist. *Br. J. Clin. Pharmacol.*, **28**, 435–41, 1989.
[2] Aellig, W.H. Nuclear magnetic resonance in clinical pharmacology and measurement of therapeutic response. *Br. J. Clin. Pharmacol.*, **29**, 157–67, 1990.
[3] Al-Sereiti, M.R., Coakes, R.L., O'Sullivan, D.P.D., and Turner, P. A comparison of the ocular hypotensive effect of 0.025% bromocriptine and 0.25% timolol eye drops in normal human volunteers. *Br. J. Clin. Pharmacol.*, **28**, 443–7, 1989.
[4] Dimenas, E., Dahlof, C., Olofsson, B., and Wiklund, I. CNS-related subjective symptoms during treatment with β_1-adrenoceptor antagonists

(atenolol, metoprolol): two double-blind placebo controlled studies. *Br. J. Clin. Pharmacol.*, **28**, 527–34, 1989.

[5] Kitchingman, G.K., Prichard, P.J., Daneshmend, T.K., Walt, R.P., and Hawkey, C.J. Enhanced gastric mucosal bleeding with doses of aspirin used for prophylaxis and its reduction by ranitidine. *Br. J. Clin. Pharmacol.*, **28**, 581–5, 1989.

[6] Lahtela, J.T. and Sotaniemi, E.A. Effect of short-acting nitroglycerin on heart rate: evaluation by a self-monitoring device. *Br. J. Clin. Pharmacol.*, **28**, 605–7, 1989.

[7] Larsson, P.T., Martinsson, A., Olsson, G., and Hjemdahl, P. Altered adrenoceptor responsiveness during adrenaline infusion, but not during mental stress: differences between receptor subtypes and tissues. *Br. J. Clin. Pharmacol.*, **28**, 663–74, 1989.

[8] Lipworth, B.J., Tregaskis, B.F., and McDevitt, D.G. β-adrenoceptor responses to inhaled salbutamol in the elderly. *Br. J. Clin. Pharmacol.*, **28**, 725–9, 1989.

[9] MacDonald, N.J., Butters, L., O'Shaughnessy, D.J., Riddell, A.J., and Rubin, P.C. A comparison of the effects of human alpha calcitonin gene-related peptide and glyceryl trinitrate on regional blood velocity in man. *Br. J. Clin. Pharmacol.*, **28**, 257–61, 1989.

[10] Petring, O.U. The effect of oxytocin on basal and pethidine-induced delayed gastric emptying. *Br. J. Clin. Pharmacol.*, **28**, 329–32, 1989.

[11] Snyman, J.R., Meyer, E.C., and Schoeman, H.S. Cimetidine as modulator of the cell-mediated immune response *in vivo* using the tuberculin skin test as parameter. *Br. J. Clin. Pharmacol.*, **29**, 257–60, 1990.

[12] Stacher, G., Gaupmann, G., Schneider, C., Stacher-Janotta, G., Steiner-Mittelbach, A., Abatzi, Th.-A., and Steinringer, H. Effects of a 5-hydroxytryptamine$_3$ receptor antagonist (CS 205–930) on colonic motor activity in healthy men. *Br. J. Clin. Pharmacol.*, **28**, 315–22, 1989.

[13] Wildin, J.D., Pleuvry, B.J., Mawer, G.E., Onon, T., and Millington, L. Respiratory and sedative effects of clobazam and clonazepam in volunteers. *Br. J. Clin. Pharmacol.*, **29**, 169–77, 1990.

17. The Use of Clinical Samples for the Biomonitoring of Genotoxic Exposure to Pharmaceutical Products

R.D. Combes

Introduction

Scope and Definitions

This paper discusses methods available and a rationale for using biomonitoring to assess the genotoxicity of medicinal products. The advantages, justification and utility of biomonitoring to detect endogenous genotoxic exposure at various stages of drug development are discussed with respect to the risk from exposure and the potential benefits from the enhanced relevance of the resulting data for predicting human hazard. A new scheme for toxicology testing of drugs, incorporating biomonitoring for genotoxicity, is presented.

Genotoxicity is the induction of DNA damage, by either covalent interaction of a chemical species with DNA (adduction) or physical alteration in the native structure of DNA. Biomonitoring (biological monitoring) is the measurement of endogenous exposure by analysis of a biological specimen or sample so as to estimate the level of a chemical, or its metabolites, within individuals at specific target sites. The information gained is used to assess the extent to which such exposures may lead to toxicity in man.[58] Monitoring for genotoxicity (*Figure 17.1*)[32,26] essentially comprises the use, in a genotoxicity assay, of clinical samples derived from a population of individuals that has been exposed to one or more potential genotoxins. Exposure can be due to occupation, diet, habit or from intentional administration of a test compound. Clinical samples can be recovered at different times following cessation of exposure to permit study of recovery due to DNA repair.

Regulatory Requirements for Pre-Clinical Testing

A scheme for drug development (*Figure 17.2*), based on current guidelines, involves a pre-clinical toxicology stage in which attempts are made to demonstrate non-genotoxicity as well as lack of acute and sub-acute toxicity. The manner in which the drug is absorbed, metabolised and excreted after administration to animals is also established. This information, together with

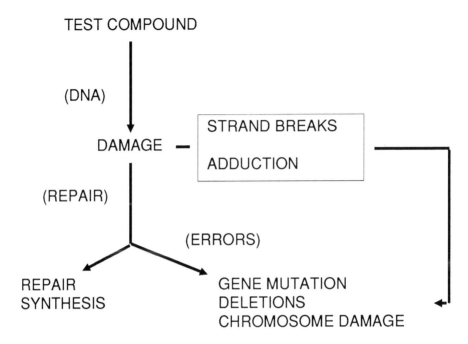

Figure 17.1. Genotoxicity end points.

details of the nature, benefits and usage of the compound, is considered prior to phase I healthy volunteer studies, comprising first administration of the drug to man.

Guidelines and regulatory requirements for the pre-clinical evaluation of the toxicology of medicinal products vary considerably worldwide. Thus, in many countries in the EEC[14], not only is there no legislation controlling volunteer studies, but also there is no official harmonisation of pre-clinical testing guidelines for phase I–II studies. One possible reason for this is a growing tendency to minimise the extent of pre-clinical toxicity required for clearance of potentially useful drugs. This is especially so with chemopreventives used for cancer and AIDS, when it is considered unethical not to undertake studies comprising first administration to man in patients at the clinical trial stage. Drug development programmes, therefore, increasingly involve human exposures at an early stage for assessment of safety and tolerance, contrary to most schemes adopted for the safety assessment of non-pharmaceutical chemicals, which rarely involve human exposure trials.

Pre-Clinical Genotoxicity Testing

Requirements for genotoxicity testing of pharmaceuticals prior to their administration to man[27] vary considerably, in both the numbers and types of tests. The majority of countries require a battery of *in vitro* and *in vivo* rodent assays deployed in a tier system approach[9], in line with widespread recommendations for the screening of chemicals for genotoxicity.[28] Assays conduc-

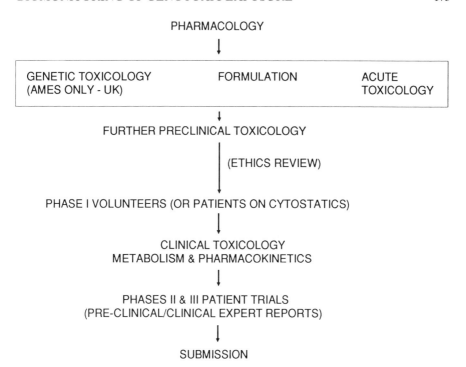

Figure 17.2. Drug development scheme.

ted *in vitro* are designed to be very sensitive in order to detect any intrinsic activity of the compound. Chemicals that are genotoxic *in vitro* are less likely to be active *in vivo*. This is because *in vitro* assays place a greater emphasis on metabolic activation, rather than detoxification, and lack mechanisms for transport of compounds/metabolites from the target site. They also remain uninfluenced by immune reactions, and suffer from the possibility of spurious data resulting from the use of high test compound concentrations and other artefactual conditions, such as excessive cytotoxicity and osmotic effects.[21,51] Thus, in tier testing schemes, *in vivo* systems are used to assess the significance of any genotoxic potential defined previously *in vitro*.

A Role for Biomonitoring

In the UK, emphasis has been placed on the use of bacterial mutation tests for pre-clinical genotoxicity of potential medicinal products.[16] Indeed, the adoption, in 1981, of a 'fast-track' system for drug development (the UK CTX scheme) essentially allows the use of only an Ames test prior to volunteer and patient studies, assuming an unequivocal negative result. This situation, in which legitimate administration of a chemical with unknown clastogenic potential to man could occur, is at variance with the reasoning underlying the strategy adopted for general screening, as not all agents which induce gene mutations are capable of causing chromosome damage. Furthermore, it is apparent that many carcinogens that go undetected by the Ames test are often positive in cytogenetics assays.[29] Thus, screening systems incorporate both a bacterial mutation assay and a test for induction of chromosomal aberrations *in vitro*. It could be argued, therefore, that it is essential to establish that an Ames negative drug is also inactive in an assay for chromosome aberrations *before* exposing healthy volunteers. In practice, this is the most likely procedure to be employed. However, for assessing human hazard, considerable advantage could be gained by utilising clinical samples, obtained during phase I and subsequent pharmacokinetic/metabolic studies for biomonitoring of genotoxicity. The results of such investigations would facilitate determination of genotoxic hazard prior to and during phase II–III clinical trials in patients. Use of biomonitoring could be considered in conjunction with, or in place of, the additional genotoxicity testing required currently by other regulatory bodies (UK and EEC)[14] as a prerequisite for product licence application.

Methods for Biomonitoring Genotoxicity

Types of Assays

A variety of clinical samples can be used, including blood, body fluids, faeces and exfoliative cells in molecular, cytogenetic and gene mutation assays (*Table 17.1*). Desirable attributes of techniques for biomonitoring include sensitivity, an ability to provide quantitative, reproducible and non-artefactual information, cheapness and rapidity.[21] In this context, sensitivity is defined as the lowest dose level of compound that can be detected

Table 17.1. Assays and samples for genotoxicity biomonitoring.*

	Blood					
	PBL	TL	RBC	Body fluids	Faeces	Exfol cells
DNA adds	Y			Y[†]		(Y)
DNA migr	Y					
Hb adds			Y			
AMES				Y	Y	
GM		Y[‡]		Y		
CA	Y			(Y)		
SCE	Y			(Y)		
UDS	Y					
MN	(Y)					Y

* Abbreviations: adds, adducts; CA, chromosome aberrations; EXFOL, exfoliative cells (e.g. urothelial/buccal cells from smokers or betel nut chewers); GM, gene mutation; Hb, haemoglobin; migr, migration; MN, micronucleus induction; PBL, peripheral blood lymphocytes; RBC, red blood cells; SCE, sister chromatid exchange; TL, T-lymphocytes; UDS, unscheduled DNA synthesis; Y, test done routinely; (Y), test theoretically possible.
† Adducts detected in urine.
‡ 6-Thioguanine resistance.
** Cultured lymphocytes.

unambiguously as active compared with background. A specific system is one providing information as to the nature of the particular endogenous exposure.[32]

Types of Clinical Samples

Blood

Blood provides a source of cells which can variously act as indicators for the measurement of molecular, cytogenetic and gene mutation endpoints (*Table 17.1*).[40] Not only can cultured lymphocytes be used, but also erythrocytes can be sampled to measure covalent binding to various sites on the haemoglobin molecule as an indirect indication of genotoxic exposure, being attributed to the endogenous generation of reactive forms of chemicals (electrophiles).[17,19,54] Blood can also be measured for systemic levels of genotoxic metabolites in the body, since serum and other cells, such as lymphocytes, circulate rapidly within the peripheral supply and throughout organs. Also, comparatively large volumes can be collected readily and repeatedly, within reasonably short periods of time from the same individual. Samples should be obtained for analysis soon after dosing, owing to eventual and often rapid transfer of most drugs from the site of administration into the circulatory system. Moreover, the data can be related to pharmacokinetic and metabolite profiles, obtained with the same samples.

Lymphocytes exist in the body for at least several years without dividing, and a proportion exhibits excessive longevity. Consequently, the study of accumulation and persistence of genotoxic damage over long periods of time, especially under conditions of repeated compound administration, is feasible. This is not so using body fluids such as urine, owing to the relatively rapid excretion of metabolites.

Sub-populations of lymphocytes exist which differ in their metabolic activation, DNA repair, immunological properties and proliferative capacity. Such phenomena, together with the presence of different distributions of chromosomal fragile sites, are thought to contribute substantially to inter- and intra-individual discrepancies observed in the responses to similar chemical exposures.[40] Erythrocytes from bone marrow have also been analysed for cytogenetic effects. However, as their collection is complicated, they have not been used widely.[23]

Body Fluids and Faeces

Several body fluids, both secretions and excretions such as urine, gastric juice, bile, nipple aspirate and perspiration, as well as serum, amniotic, peritoneal and other fluids, may be utilised, although obviously these vary in the degree of invasiveness involved in their collection.[13,59] Faecal stool samples have also been used.[59]

Body fluid and faecal analyses differ from other methods for biomonitoring in that they do not entail detection of the genotoxic event in human cells recovered from an individual after exposure, but rather involve the same indicators, such as bacteria and cultured mammalian cells, that are used in conventional assays. Thus, the use of such human fluids still suffers from several of the drawbacks of *in vitro* assays, especially the lack of an immune response and transport of metabolites away from the target site.

Despite non-invasive and easy collection of most fluids, their utilisation has several other disadvantages.[59] These include a frequent need for complicated concentration and extraction techniques to obtain sufficient concentrations of metabolites free from interfering substances which may give spurious effects. Negative data may therefore result from inefficient extraction methods.[13] Extracts may also be labile during storage and may require enzymatic deconjugation.

Body fluid and faecal analyses are extremely sensitive to complicating factors such as diet, occupation, lifestyle and other exposures, as well as to changes in sample collection time, all of which combine to confound data interpretation.[59] Attempts have been made to overcome the problems of variable composition of urine samples by standardising the data with respect to creatinine levels. A further confounding factor in the interpretation of body fluid assays is a frequent need for further activation *in vitro*, a feature which is contrary to the rationale underlying body fluid analysis to overcome the problems of using exogenous metabolising systems. Moreover, administration of a genotoxic compound that is not absorbed may result in active or inactive extracts depending on the sample used.[13,36]

A major advantage of assays using excretions such as urine is the possibility of relating genotoxicity data to the results of concurrent metabolite analyses in order to assist in data interpretation. In addition, detection of thioethers in urine is an indication of endogenous generation of reactive forms of chemicals (electrophiles).[24] These arise when activated intermediates are conjugated with glutathione.

Exfoliative Cells
Studies with exfoliative cells have been limited to the study of smokers and betal nut chewers using cytogenetic assays with urothelial and buccal samples, respectively.[32,46]

Selection of Samples

The choice of clinical sample is limited by a need for sampling to be as non-invasive as possible. Also, factors such as the nature of the drug, the intended route of administration and action, and its known or suspected biological fate, should be considered when selecting samples. Thus, if the aim is to study endogenous causes of a particular cancer, of the stomach or breast for example, then it would be appropriate to analyse gastric juice or nipple aspirate, respectively, for mutagenic metabolites. Relevant tissue-specific secretions can be used in each situation.[13] Indeed, it has been argued[6] that target tissue cytology, assessed by studies of the cytogenetics of appropriate exfoliative cells, will provide the most useful data for assessing potential carcinogenic hazard. However, it is likely that the most relevant indication of possible endogenous genotoxic exposure will be derived from blood collected for biomonitoring of new drugs. The testing of urinary extracts for the presence of mutagenic and clastogenic metabolites, utilising a variety of genotoxic endpoints in conjunction with metabolism data, may also be a useful adjunctive approach in certain circumstances.

Genotoxic Endpoints

Overview
Several reviews provide an introduction to and detailed discussion of geno-toxicity and the methods involved in the major assays.[60,62] Endpoints that can be measured using biomonitoring and their inter-relationships are shown in *Figure 17.1*. If an exposure induces DNA damage, such as adduction, base alteration or nucleotide strand breakage, the cell responds by attempting to repair the lesion and to restore the former, native DNA structure. Repair can fail or mistakes can occur during the process (error-prone repair), leading to alterations in base sequence and possibly gene mutation. Larger effects, perhaps also due to a loss of nucleotides (deletion), can culminate in structural damage to chromosomes, such as breakage (clastogenesis).

Interaction with DNA (adduction) can be measured directly using several molecular techniques, while other methods are available for detecting the consequences of such interaction in terms of repair, gene mutation and chromosome damage.

DNA adducts
Procedures for monitoring DNA adduction may be divided into those suitable for the measurement of adducts and others designed to permit adduct characterisation.[43,64] DNA binding requires the availability and use of a radioactive test compound,[15] which should not necessarily be a limitation during pre-clinical testing of drugs. However, association of radio-label with extracted DNA could be due to metabolic recycling and incorporation via the nucleotide pool. Thus, it is necessary to demonstrate the presence of adducts using chromatography.

^{32}P-postlabelling does not utilise radio-labelled test material. After treatment, DNA is purified, hydrolysed to its component, single nucleosides, and phosphorylated with high specific activity ^{32}P. Adducted nucleosides are separated from unaltered ones by TLC or HPLC and assayed by scintillation counting. Recent modifications to these methods have extended the range of detectable bulky and non-bulky adducts. Limited identification of adducts can be achieved by this approach. However, they can be characterised more fully using analytical chemistry and immunoassay with poly- and monoclonal antibodies.[61,63] In practice, however, such methods are complicated and unsuitable for routine biomonitoring, since availability of standards and specific antisera is essential.

Molecular techniques are extremely sensitive with detection varying from 1 adduct in 10^6 to 1 in 10^{10} nucleosides. They may be used to detect induction of DNA damage in peripheral blood lymphocytes, and also the excretion of adducted nucleosides in the peripheral blood lymphocytes and urine of patients, respectively.[45]

DNA damage can be measured in individual lymphocytes using microgel electrophoresis,[53] by embedding the cells in agarose gel on a microscope slide and subjecting them to detergent/high salt concentration lysis under alkaline conditions. The DNA is electrophoresed in alkali and damage is scored by measuring the extent of migration (in mm) from the cell nucleus to the anode after ethidium bromide staining and fluorescence determination. Both double- and single-strand breaks can be detected as a result of nucleotide strand unwinding at high pH. However, this sensitive technique is probably more suited to investigating differences in individual susceptibilities to various exposures, rather than for routine biomonitoring.

DNA Repair

A decrease in genotoxicity with increasing time between exposure and sampling in any assay can be taken as an indication of DNA repair, assuming that the change is due to removal of DNA damage.

The extent of repair can be measured directly as 'unscheduled DNA synthesis' (UDS). UDS involves measurement, by ^{3}H-thymidine autoradiography, or scintillation counting, of the small amount of DNA synthesis that occurs in otherwise non-replicating DNA within non-dividing cells, as a result of replacement of a small portion of a nucleotide strand bearing the lesion which was enzymatically excised. UDS can be undertaken using lymphocytes, although it is considered unlikely to be a sensitive indicator of endogenous, genotoxic exposure.[22]

Gene Mutation

Of the few available, established *in vivo* assays for measuring somatic gene mutation, the detection of variants of T-lymphocytes in peripheral blood, which are resistant to the purine analogue 6-thioguanine (6-TG), has been used extensively for biomonitoring.[2,3] Resistance is acquired by a mutation in the hypoxanthine phosphoribosyl-transferase (HGPRT) gene that abolishes the conversion of 6-TG to a toxic nucleotide which is incorporated into DNA. 6-TG^r cells are selected in medium containing the analogue and counted either by autoradiography or by cloning.

Cytogenetics

Chromosome damage is one of the most extensively used endpoints for human genotoxic biomonitoring[18], and involves scoring chromosomal and nuclear alterations mainly in peripheral blood lymphocytes of exposed individuals.[10,50] Structural effects, due to direct breakage and chromosomal rearrangements, are recorded, as well as sister chromatid exchanges (SCE) due to intrachromosomal events, involving symmetrical exchanges, which occur along the chromosome by some, as yet obscure, mechanism.

Micronuclei are also scored. Each micronucleus is a portion of chromatin surrounded by a separate nuclear membrane which arises in one of two ways – condensation of acentric chromosomes that remain separate at anaphase owing to their inability to attach to the spindle at cell division, or exclusion of intact, centric chromosomes from anaphase segregation as a consequence of spindle disruption. Thus, the existence of increased numbers of micronuclei is evidence of prior induction of chromosomal damage, or of a potential, indirect alteration of the genome caused by non-disjunction (aberrant chromosome segregation). Since a growing number of carcinogens is being demonstrated as acting by such non-genotoxic mechanisms, centromere-specific antibodies are being used to differentiate between the two types of micronuclei.[25]

Detection of micronuclei in peripheral blood arising as a consequence of *in vivo* exposure is compromised as the spleen serves to remove micronucleated cells. However, increases in micronucleated peripheral blood erythrocytes have been observed, following treatment of splenectomised individuals with various anti-cancer drugs.[49] As an alternative to this unsuitable method for routine biomonitoring, micronuclei can be assessed in cultured binucleated lymphocytes, using a cytochalasin-B technique to block cytokinesis, so that a sub-population of cells that have recently undergone nuclear division subsequent to exposure can be defined.[20]

Comparison of Methods

Molecular methods of biomonitoring are more sensitive and, in some cases, more specific for particular types of DNA damage than cytogenetics assays. The major reason for this relates to the fact that exposed cells first have to undergo DNA replication for chemically induced DNA lesions to be manifest as chromosome damage leading to aberrations, micronuclei or SCEs. This process is hindered for two reasons. Firstly, lymphocytes persist in the blood for long periods without dividing and there is adequate time for repair. Secondly, cells are continually being removed from the circulating blood. However, molecular techniques require sophisticated instrumentation, and their inherent high sensitivity complicates data interpretation owing to the frequent detection of high background levels of genotoxicity in unexposed individuals. On the other hand, chromosomal analysis requires a microscope and tissue-culturing facilities. Nevertheless, experienced staff are needed for the time-consuming process of scoring. However, these are considerations which apply whether biomonitoring or *in vitro* assays are being performed.

SCEs and micronuclei are easier to identify than aberrations[55], although visualisation of the former requires a more complicated procedure than that necessary to detect the other two classes of cytogenetic damage. SCEs occur more frequently after treatments with low dose levels of a wide range of chemicals, especially those causing DNA adducts, although only modest levels of SCE induction occurred following various exposures, including anti-cancer drug therapy.[11,22] However, certain clastogens are unable to induce SCEs and exchange formation relies on the presence of a lesion at replication. Nevertheless, it is likely that SCE analysis of peripheral lymphocytes will continue to be a widely used method for biomonitoring.[6,7]

Image analysis and immunochemical labelling of chromosomes are now being used to facilitate cytogenetic analysis of both structural and numerical changes in the karyotype.[36,42,44]

Potential Problems with Biomonitoring Assays

Many of the factors complicating data interpretation are beyond the control of the investigator. However, their potential influence on the results can often be minimised by using the same individuals to provide baseline control data. This is achieved by analysing samples before treatment, as well as after a recovery period following cessation of dosing, a common practice during pre-clinical toxicology. Some individuals may be unsuitable for this form of biomonitoring owing to excessively high background levels and/or sample variation in genotoxic activity. Inter-individual variation, both in the background levels of genotoxicity in cells from unexposed subjects and in cells from subjects given identical treatments, has been recorded frequently.[4,23,31] This complicates data interpretation and necessitates the use of large numbers of donors to improve the power of statistical analysis.

Examples of Biomonitoring from the Literature

Extensive use has been made of cytogenetic analysis for surveillance of human populations subjected to occupational exposures in the work place.[7] Most studies on exposure to medicinal compounds, especially those demonstrating genotoxic exposure, have involved lymphocytes from individuals, including patients, receiving chemotherapy (*Tables 17.2* and *17.3*). The reader is referred to Gebhart's extensive review of the literature and discussion of problems associated with cytogenetics monitoring.[23] His database cites 110 different chemotherapeutic agents, of which half unequivocally increased the incidence of cytogenetic abnormalities. These were scored primarily as chromosomal aberrations, less as SCEs and very few as micronuclei.

In many cases, the data exhibited close agreement with the results of *in vitro* and animal genotoxicity assays. However, there are several compounds which proved inactive after therapeutic exposures to humans, but positive in

Table 17.2. Some genotoxic drugs and related compounds subjected to biomonitoring assays.*

Compound	Sample	Assay	Group	Reference
cis-Platinum	PBL	IA	Cancer patients	45
16 Cytostatics	PBL	CA	Cancer patients,	30
		SCE	nurses	
	Urine	AMES		
Cytostatics	PB(T-L)	GM	Nurses	2
	EC/EB	MN	Leukaemia patients	1
Cyclophosphamide	PBL	CA	Manufacturing and/or	56
		SCE	packaging workers,	
	Urine	AMES	nurses	
	PB(T-L)	GM	MS patients	3
	Urine	AMES	Patients	56
Cytostatics*	Sweat	AMES	Cancer patients	34
Coal tar (pure	PBL	CA/SCE	Psoriasis patients	47
or 4%)	Urine	AMES[†]		
	PB(T-L)	GM		2
Nitrofurantoin	Urine	AMES	Patients	59
niridazole				
Bleomycin	EC	SCE	Cancer patients	11
Cimetidine/NO$_2$	GJ	AMES	Patients	59

* Abbreviations: CA, chromosomal aberrations; EB, erythroblasts; EC, erythrocytes; GJ, gastric juice; GM, gene mutation (6-TG resistance); IA, immunoassay; PBL, peripheral blood lymphocytes; PB(T-L), T-lymphocytes.
† Various mixtures of cyclophosphamide, vinblastine and phenylalanine mustard.
‡ Polycyclic aromatic hydrocarbons in urine.

Table 17.3. Some non-genotoxic drugs and related compounds subjected to biomonitoring assays.*

Compound	Sample	Assay	Group	Reference
Phenobarbitone	PBL	SCE	Epilepsy patients	48
Feverfew	PBL	CA	Migraine patients	5
	Urine	AMES		
Sodium selenite	PBL	CA	Cancer patients	39
		SCE		
Cyclophosphamide	PBL	CA	Manufacturing and/or	56
		SCE	packaging workers,	
	Urine	AMES	nurses	

* CA, chromosomal aberrations; PBL, peripheral blood lymphocytes.

conventional testing.[23] An example is sodium selenite, which induced aberrations in rat lymphocytes *in vitro*, but not in lymphocytes of patients given injections or tablets (<0.05 mg/kg daily for 1–13 months). The chemical was, however, active in the bone marrow of rats, but not in lymphocytes from the same species,[38,39] possibly because of differences between the longevity and repair status of the respective indicator cells.

The results[30] of cytogenetic analysis of peripheral blood from five non-smoking cancer patients receiving a variety of drug cocktails are shown in *Figure 17.3*. Increases in genotoxicity are apparent in all cases when scored as

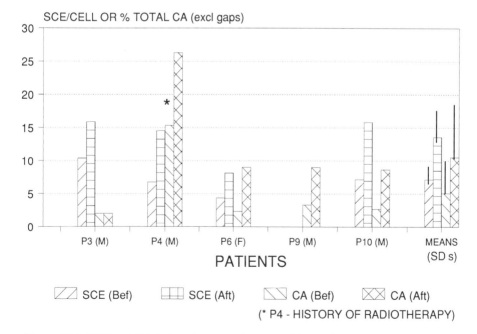

Figure 17.3. SCE and CA in lymphocytes of non-smoking patients on cytostatic drugs. (Adapted from Krepinsky *et al.*, 1990.[30])

SCEs, but not when aberrations were recorded. Differences in susceptibilities to treatment and in background frequencies of damage generate non-significant differences when the mean values for this small population are compared. The high incidence of aberrations in patient 4 was attributed to a history of radiotherapy. These results illustrate the susceptibility of biomonitoring to confounding factors and the problems of inter-individual variability mentioned earlier.

Krepinsky et al.[30] and several other investigators (Table 17.2) have observed substantial levels of endogenous genotoxic exposure of nurses and associated personnel who handle chemotherapeutic agents and other drugs. This phenomenon has also been demonstrated in some hospital operating staff when thioethers, but not mutagens, have been detected in their urine after exposure to anaesthetics.[41] Such observations imply that patients, although the intended targets, are not the only population potentially at risk from exposure to drugs. In addition, other routes of administration, such as dermal, should be considered, where appropriate, when designing biomonitoring studies. Genotoxic analysis may also prove useful in monitoring the success of improvements in techniques and safety precautions for handling drugs.[56]

In contrast with the situation with chemopreventives, few studies have been conducted with other drugs and related compounds, and most of these have yielded evidence for non-genotoxicity (Tables 17.2 and 17.3).

Rationale for Using Biomonitoring

Advantages and Justification

In addition to the deficiencies of in vitro assays discussed above, these systems are likely to be unsuitable for testing large molecular weight compounds such as biotechnology-derived protein products. There is a high chance that the data obtained will be spurious as a result of a lack of cellular uptake of the compound, or of the induction of damage to membranes of cells in tissue culture. Some of these products, e.g. hormones, may exert indirect effects which will only occur in vivo, and selection of the most appropriate assay needs careful consideration. Many biotechnology-derived products will be immunogenic, and this activity may compromise toxicity determination in animals,[8] necessitating human studies.

There are several justifications for the adoption of a role for human biomonitoring, in place of, or as an adjunct to, animal genotoxicity studies, for confirmation and clarification of results of in vitro assays. Firstly, exposure to drugs is primarily intentional. Secondly, no animal model will simulate accurately all the processes which determine toxicity to man. Such toxicity may be expected with chemicals that are designed specifically to exert biological activity within the body.[52] Moreover, drug efficacy can be fully established only from controlled dosing studies using humans.

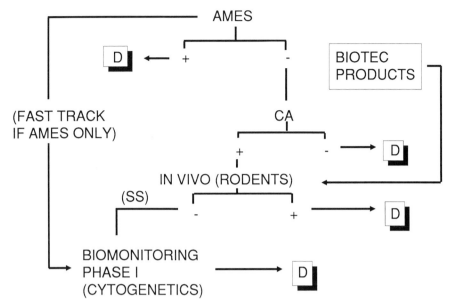

Figure 17.4. Proposed scheme for genotoxicity testing of drugs. D = decision point, SS = species specificity, CA = chromosomal aberrations.

Recommendations

Proposed Scheme

A suggested tier-testing scheme (*Figure 17.4*) involves initial screening for bacterial mutation, followed by testing non-mutagens for chromosomal aberrations in cultured mammalian cells. Compounds which remain non-genotoxic could then be assessed using rodent systems *in vivo*, as undertaken for non-pharmaceutical chemicals. At each stage, decisions on whether to proceed with development will need to take into account the data obtained and other factors, such as the nature of the drug, its intended usage and the potential resulting benefits. The timing and extent of other *in vitro* tests, animal assays and biomonitoring in the scheme will depend upon scientific, ethical and risk-benefit considerations.

It is likely that the majority of candidate drugs will be subjected to Ames testing and *in vitro* cytogenetics at a very early stage in product development. Genotoxicity in either or both of these tests should not necessarily preclude further evaluation, especially in the case of marginal, weak or inconsistent, potentially artefactual situations. Moreover, there may be an urgent thera-peutic need for the compound. There is also a requirement for continued testing of anti-neoplastics, whose cytostatic activities will be dependent upon interaction with DNA, with the consequent high chance of genotoxicity and carcinogenicity.[33]

Other Considerations

The deficiencies of animal assays, arising from many factors, including age- and species-dependent metabolism, and differences in bioavailability, are increased when animals of uniform age and inappropriate routes or excessively high dose levels are used.[35] Early utilisation of human studies, in conjunction with genotoxicity assays, is recommended to overcome many of these shortcomings, especially when species-specificity in response is known or suspected. If a rapid pre-clinical testing scheme is adopted in which genotoxicity is limited to Ames testing, biomonitoring should involve an assessment of cytogenetic effects. Volunteer studies usually involve administration of single ascending doses starting at a very low level. Evidence for genotoxicity can be sought at each dose level, especially as several of the assays are highly sensitive. After administration of several, increasing doses, it should be possible to define values for no- or minimal-effect levels, and to obtain dose responses in order to facilitate data interpretation, within the limits of therapeutic exposures. Further clarification of potential safety may be forthcoming from the analysis of samples collected at different times after dosing, to detect recovery and repair.

A study of drug activity in diseased individuals obviously has to be deferred until efficacy trials (phases II and III), as healthy volunteers are frequently used in phase I. Specific effects can be investigated at these later stages, depending on previous data and the clinical uses of the drug. For example, potential toxicity to germ cells or to the foetus (by a compound intended for use during pregnancy) can be determined by analysis of sperm abnormality or by cytogenetic analysis of cord blood and foetal tissue.[12,32] In addition, evaluation of DNA adduction at various tissue sites permits assessment of the efficacy of cytostatics under clinical conditions. There is also a need to expand the nature of post-market surveillance, in view of the substantial number of reported cases of adverse reactions to drugs[57], and worthwhile improvements in surveillance could be achieved by continuing to study genotoxicity using clinical samples.

Conclusions

It is perhaps surprising that biomonitoring for genotoxicity has not been more widely used and advocated in the safety evaluation of drugs, especially in view of calls for more extensive utilisation of volunteers and occupationally exposed groups for assessing toxicity of industrial chemicals.[26] It is essential that biomonitoring be applied judiciously for two main reasons. Firstly, limitations of assays should be considered, when designing studies, to allow sufficient sampling to alleviate the effects of several confounding factors. Larger numbers of individuals than for conventional volunteer and patient studies may be required to achieve this, although the same controlled conditions and, preferably, the same clinical samples should be used to enable direct comparison of the different data obtained. Secondly, it is necessary to consider all of the available information relating to any particular drug, so as to minimise the risk of human exposure at all stages of safety assessment. However, the level of risk should be assessed in relation to the size of the population exposure required for the study, the potential reliability and predictive value of the resulting information, and the benefits to society of the product in question.

It is to be hoped that adoption of the above rationale will result in more extensive usage of clinical samples for analysis of genotoxicity in the safety assessment of pharmaceutical products. The enhanced relevance of the information obtained, with respect to predicting human hazard, should not deter consideration of this approach in the pharmaceutical industry.

Acknowledgements

The author is grateful to A. Cameron, L.M. Holmstrom and A.B. Wilson for comments on the manuscript.

References

[1] Abe, T., Isemura, T., and Kikuchi, Y. Micronuclei in human bone marrow cells: evaluation of the micronucleus test using human leukaemia patients treated with antileukaemic agents. *Mutation Res.*, **130**, 113–20, 1984.

[2] Albertini, R.J. Studies with T-lymphocytes: an approach to human mutagenicity monitoring. In *Indicators of Genotoxic Exposure*, Banbury Report No. 13, Cold Spring Harbor Laboratory, New York, pp 393–412, 1982.

[3] Ammenheuser, M.M., Ward, Jr., J.B., Whorton, E.B., Killian, J.M., and Legator, M.S. Elevated frequencies of 6-thioguanine-resistant lymphocytes in multiple sclerosis patients treated with cyclophosphamide: a prospective study. *Mutation Res.*, **204**, 509–20, 1988.

[4] Anderson, D. (ed). Human biomonitoring. *Mutation Res.*, **204**, 353–551, 1988.

[5] Anderson, D., Jenkinson, P.C., Dewdney, R.S., Blowers, S.D., Johnson, E.S., and Kadam, N.P. Chromosomal aberrations and sister chromatid exchanges in lymphocytes and urine mutagenicity of migraine patients: a comparison of chronic feverfew users and matched non-users. *Human Toxicol.*, **7**, 145–52, 1988.

[6] Ashby, J. Comparison of techniques for monitoring human exposure to genotoxic chemicals. *Mutation Res.*, **204**, 543–51, 1988.

[7] Ashby, J. and Richardson, C.R. Tabulation and assessment of 113 human surveillance cytogenetic studies conducted between 1965 and 1984. *Mutation Res.*, **154**, 111–33, 1985.

[8] Bangham, D.R. 'New biological products' and toxicity tests. In *Advances in Applied Toxicology*, A.D. Dyan and A.J.Paine (eds), pp 133–42, Taylor and Francis, London, 1989.

[9] Bridges, B.A. Genetic toxicology at the crossroads: a personal view on the deployment of short-term tests for predicting carcinogenicity. *Mutation Res.*, **205**, 25–32, 1988.

[10] Carrano, A.V. and Natarajan, A.T. Considerations for population monitoring using cytogenetic techniques. *Mutation Res.*, **204**, 379–406, 1988.

[11] Clare, M.G., Taylor, J.H., Blain, E., and Jones, W.G. The quantitation of sister chromatid exchanges in lymphocytes of cancer patients at intervals after cytostatic chemotherapy. *Eur. J. Cancer Clin. Oncol.*, **19**, 1509–15, 1983.

[12] Cole, R.J. and Henderson, L. Measuring prenatal genotoxic effects in mice and men. In *Indicators of Genotoxic Exposure* Banbury Report No. 13, Cold Spring Harbor Laboratory, New York, pp 355–67, 1982.

[13] Combes, R.D., Anderson, D., Brooks, T., Neale, S., and Venitt, S. Mutagens in urine, faeces and body fluids. In *Report of the UKEMS Sub-committee on Guidelines for Mutagenicity Testing, Part II: Supplementary Tests; Mutagens in Food; Mutagens in Body Fluids and Excreta; Nitrosation Products*, B.J. Dean (ed), UKEMS, Swansea, UK, pp 203–43, 1984.

[14] Commission of the European Community. *The Rules Governing Medicinal Products in the European Community, Volume III: Guidelines on the Quality, Safety and Efficacy of Medicinal Products for Human Use*, EEC, Brussels, 1989.

[15] Dashwood, R.H. and Combes, R.D. Deficiencies in the covalent binding index (CBI) for expressing *in vivo* binding to DNA with respect to predicting chemical carcinogenicity. A proposal for a target organ binding index. *Mutation Res.*, **190**, 173–5, 1987.

[16] Department of Health and Social Security. *Medicines Act 1968. Guidance Notes on Applications for Clinical Trials Certificates and Clinical Trial Exemptions*. HMSO, London, 1986.

[17] European Chemical Industry Ecology and Toxicology Centre (ECETOX). *DNA and protein adducts: evaluation of their use in exposure monitoring and risk assessment. No. 13,* ECETOX, Brussels, Belgium, 1987.

[18] Evans, H.J. Mutation cytogenetics: past, present and future. *Mutation Res.*, **204**, 355–63, 1988.

[19] Farmer, P.B., Neumann, H-G., and Henschler, D. Estimation of exposure of man to substances reacting covalently with macromolecules. *Arch. Toxicol.*, **60**, 251–60, 1987.

[20] Fenech, M. and Morley, A.A. Solutions to the kinetic problem in the micronucleus assay. *Cytobios*, **43**, 223–46, 1985.

[21] Galloway, S.M., Deasy, D.A., Bean, C.L., Kraynak, A.R., Armstrong, M.J., and Bradley, M.O. Effects of high osmotic strength on chromosome aberrations, sister chromatid exchanges and DNA strand breaks, and their relation to toxicity. *Mutation Res.*, **189**, 15–25, 1987.

[22] Garner, R.C. Assessment of carcinogen exposure in man. *Carcinogenesis*, **6**, 1071–8, 1985.

[23] Gebhart, E. Chromosomal aberrations in lymphocytes of patients under chemotherapy. In *Mutations in Man*, G. Obe (ed), pp 198–222, Springer-Verlag, Berlin, 1984.

[24] Henderson, P.T., Van Doorn, R., Leijdekkers, C-M., and Bos, R.P. Excretion of thioethers in the urine after exposure to electrophilic chemicals. In *Monitoring Human Exposure to Carcinogenic and Mutagenic Agents,* IARC Scientific Publications No. 59, A. Berlin, M. Draper, K. Hemminki, and H. Vainio (eds), pp 173–88, IARC, Lyon, 1984.

[25] Hennig, U.G.G., Rudd, N.L., and Hoar, D.I. Kinetochore immunofluorescence in micronuclei: a rapid method for the *in situ* detection of aneuploidy and chromosome breakage in human fibroblasts. *Mutation Res.*, **203**, 405–14, 1988.

[26] Howe, W., Stonard, M.D., and Woollen, B.H. The use of human biological measurements for safety evaluation in the chemical industry. In *The Future of Predictive Safety Evaluation*, Vol. 1, A.N. Worden, D.V. Parke, and J. Marks (eds), pp 63–78, MTP Press Ltd., Lancaster, UK, 1986.

[27] Inveresk Research International. *Regulatory Affairs Guidelines No. 5: Genetic Toxicity*, IRI Ltd., Tranent, Scotland, 1990.

[28] Ishidate Jr., M. A proposed battery of tests for the initial evaluation of the mutagenic potential of medicinal and industrial chemicals. *Mutation Res.*, **205**, 397–407, 1988.

[29] Ishidate Jr., M., Harnois, M.C., and Sofuni, T. A comparative analysis of data on the clastogenicity of 951 chemical substances tested in mammalian cell cultures. *Mutation Res.*, **195**, 151–213, 1988.

[30] Krepinsky, A., Bryant, D.W., Davison, L., Young, B., Heddle, J., McCalla, D.R., Douglas, G., and Michalko, K. Comparison of three assays for genetic effects of antineoplasic drugs on cancer patients and their nurses. *Environ. Molecular Mutagenesis*, **15**, 83–92, 1990.

[31] Leonard, A. Cytogenetic observations in human somatic cells. In *Indicators for Assessing Exposure and Biological Effects of Genotoxic Chemicals*, A. Aitio, G. Becking, A. Berlin, A. Bernard, V. Foa, D. Kello, E. Krug, A. Leonard, and G. Nordberg (eds), pp 83–138, Commission of the European Communities, Brussels, 1988.

[32] Lohmann, P.H.M., Jansen, J.D., and Baan, R. Comparison of various methodologies with respect to specificity and sensitivity in biomonitoring occupational exposure to mutagens and carcinogens. In *Monitoring Human Exposure to Carcinogenic and Mutagenic Agents*, IARC Scientific Publications No. 59, A. Berlin, M. Draper, K. Hemminki, and H. Vainio (eds), pp 259–77, Lyon, IARC, 1984.

[33] Ludlum, D.B. Therapeutic agents as potential carcinogens. In *Chemical Carcinogenesis and Mutagenesis*, Vol.1, C.S. Cooper and P.L. Grover (eds), pp 153–75, 1990.

[34] Madsen, E.S. and Larsen, H. Excretion of mutagens in sweat from humans treated with antineoplastic drugs. *Cancer Lett.*, **40**, 199–202, 1988.

[35] Marks, J. Toxicology for pharmaceutical substances: the needs. In *The Future of Predictive Safety Evaluation*, Vol. 2, A.N. Worden, D.V. Parke, and J. Marks (eds), pp 245–54, MTP Press Ltd., Lancaster, UK, 1987.

[36] McGregor, D.B. Summary report on the performance of the miscellaneous group of *in vivo* assays. In *Evaluation of Short-term Tests for Carcinogens*, Vol. 2, J. Ashby, *et al.* (eds), Cambridge University Press, pp 3–21, 1988.

[37] Merry, D.E., Pathak, S., Hsu, T.C., and Brinkley, B.R. Antikinetochore antibodies: use as probes for inactive centromeres. *Amer. J. Human Genetics*, **37**, 425–30, 1985.

[38] Newton, M.F. and Lilley, L.J. Tissue-specific clastogenic effects of chromium and selenium salts *in vivo*. *Mutation Res.*, **169**, 61–9, 1986.

[39] Norppa, H., Westermark, T., Laasonen, M., Knuutila, K., and Knuutila, S. Chromosomal effects of sodium selenite *in vivo*, aberrations and sister chromatid exchanges in human lymphocytes. *Hereditas*, **93**, 93–6, 1980.

[40] Obe, G. and Beek, B. Human peripheral lymphocytes in mutation research. In *Mutations in Man*, G. Obe (ed), pp 177–97, Springer-Verlag, Berlin, 1984.

[41] Pasquini, R., Monarca, S., Scassellati Sforzolini, G., Bauleo, F.A., Angeli, G., and Cerami, F. Thioethers, mutagens, and D-glucaric acid in urine of operating room personnel exposed to anaesthetics. *Teratogen. Carcinogen. Mutagen.*, **9**, 359–68, 1989.

[42] Peretti, D., Maraschio, P., Lambiase, S., Lo Curto, F., and Zuffardi, O. Indirect immunofluorescence of inactive centromeres as indicator of centromeric function. *Human Genetics*, **73**, 12–16, 1986.

[43] Phillips, D.H. Modern methods of DNA adduct determination. In *Chemical Carcinogenesis and Mutagenesis*, Vol. 1, C.S. Cooper and P.L. Grover (eds), pp 503–46, 1990.

[44] Piper, J. and Lundsteen, C. Human chromosome analysis by machine. *Trends in Genetics*, **3**, 309–13, 1987.

[45] Poirier, M.C., Reed, E., Zwelling, L.A., Ozols, R.F., Litterst, C.L., and Yuspa, S.H. Polyclonal antibodies to quantitate cis-diamminedichloroplatinum (II)-DNA adducts in cancer patients and animal models. *Environ. Health Perspectives*, **62**, 89–94, 1985.

[46] Reali, D., Di Marino, F., Bahramandpour, S., Carducci, A., Barale, R., and Loprieno, N. Micronuclei in exfoliated urothelial cells and urine mutagenicity in smokers. *Mutation Res.*, **192**, 145–9, 1987.

[47] Sarto, F., Zordan, M., Tomanin, R., Mazzotti, D., Canova, A., Cardin, E.L., Bezze, G., and Levis, A.G. Chromosomal alterations in peripheral blood lymphocytes, urinary mutagenicity and excretion of polycyclic aromatic hydrocarbons in six psoriatic patients undergoing coal tar therapy. *Carcinogenesis*, **10**, 329–34, 1989.

[48] Schaumann, B.A., Winge, V.B., and Pederson, M. Genotoxicity evaluation in patients on phenobarbital monotherapy by sister chromatid exchange. *J. Toxicol. Environ. Health*, **28**, 277–84, 1989.

[49] Schlegel, R., MacGregor, J.T., and Everson, R.B. Assessment of cytogenetic damage by quantitation of micronuclei in human peripheral blood erythrocytes. *Cancer Res.*, **46**, 3717–21, 1986.

[50] Scott, D., Dean, B.J., Kirkland, D.J., and Danford, N. Metaphase chromosome aberration assays *in vitro*. In *Basic Mutagenicity Tests UKEMS Recommended Procedures*, D.J. Kirkland (ed.), pp 62–86, Cambridge University Press, Cambridge, UK, 1990.

[51] Seerberg, A.H., Mosesso, P., and Forster, R. High-dose-level effects in mutagenicity assays utilising mammalian cells in culture. *Mutagenesis*, **3**, 213–18, 1988.

[52] Shephard, N.W. Predictive safety evaluation: the clinical trial. In *The Future of Predictive Safety Evaluation*, Vol. 2, A.N. Worden, D.V. Parke, and J. Marks (eds), pp 255–62, MTP Press Ltd., Lancaster, UK, 1987.

[53] Singh, N.P., McCoy, M.T., Tice, R.R., and Schneider, E.L. A simple technique for quantitation of low levels of DNA damage in single cells. *Experimental Cell Res.*, **175**, 184–91, 1988.

[54] Skipper, P.L. and Tannenbaum, S.R. Protein adducts in the molecular dosimetry of chemical carcinogens. *Carcinogenesis*, **11**, 507–18, 1990.

[55] Sorsa, M. Monitoring of sister chromatid exchange and micronuclei as biological end-points. In *Monitoring Human Exposure to Carcinogenic and Mutagenic Agents*, IARC Scientific Publications No. 59, A. Berlin, M. Draper, K. Hemminki, and H. Vainio (eds), pp 339–49, Lyon, IARC, 1984.

[56] Sorsa, M., Pyy, L., Salomaa, S., Nylaund, L., and Yager, J.W. Biological and environmental monitoring of occupational exposure to cyclophosphamide in industry and hospitals. *Mutation Res.*, **204**, 465–80, 1988.

[57] Teeling-Smith, G. Economic aspects of toxicity for the pharmaceutical industry. In *The Future of Predictive Safety Evaluation*, Vol. 1, A.N. Worden, D.V. Parke, and J. Marks (eds), pp 79–87, MTP Press Ltd, Lancaster, UK, 1986.

[58] Van Sittert, N.J. Biomonitoring of chemicals and their metabolites. In

Monitoring Human Exposure to Carcinogenic and Mutagenic Agents, IARC Scientific Publications No. 59, A. Berlin, M. Draper, K. Hemminki, and H. Vainio (eds), pp 153–72, Lyon, IARC, 1984.

[59] Venitt, S. The use of short-term tests for the detection of genotoxic activity in body fluids and excreta. *Mutation Res.*, **205**, 331–53, 1988.

[60] Venitt, S. and Parry, J.M. (eds), *Mutagenicity Testing – A Practical Approach*. IRL Press Ltd., Oxford.

[61] Weston, A., Manchester, D.K., Povey, A., and Harris, C.C. Detection of carcinogen-macromolecular adducts in humans. *J. Amer. Coll. Toxicol.*, **8**, 913–32, 1989.

[62] Williams, G.M. Methods for evaluating chemical genotoxicity. *Ann. Rev. Pharmacol. Toxicol.*, **29**, 189–211, 1989.

[63] Wogan, G.N. Markers of exposure to carcinogens: methods for human biomonitoring. *J. Amer. Coll. Toxicol.*, **8**, 871–81, 1989.

18. Quality Control of New Methods of Clinical Measurement: Software and Data Handling

A. Pidgen

Introduction

Clinical measurements recorded during the lifetime of a drug are many and varied. The type of response obtained will depend largely upon the intended therapeutic use for the drug and the nature of the clinical trial being undertaken. Clinical measurements fall into two broad categories, namely *quantitative (numerical) measurements* and *qualitative (descriptive) measurements*.

A drug's development cycle encompasses a whole range of pre-clinical and clinical studies. By the time a drug is submitted for registration, well over a million measurements and/or observations will have been recorded. Therefore, accurate and efficient methods of data collection, storage, analysis and presentation are important in order to ensure a rapid development of promising drugs and an early termination of the development of poor drugs.

Computers are playing an increasingly important role in both industry and academia. Many pharmaceutical companies have some form of clinical trials database within which data are stored from clinical trials. Data entry is usually performed manually (via the keyboard), semi-automatically (via floppy disk or magnetic tape) or automatically (direct from the instrument). Direct data entry has increased in popularity over recent years to such an extent that many of the instruments currently available for use in clinics and laboratories have some form of built-in, or add-on, computer facilities for data capture and/or data processing. Robot systems have been developed for use in laboratories, where they can perform such repetitive tasks as sample tube handling in routine assay work. The scope and range of computer software are continually being expanded, and a number of 'expert' systems are now being used in such areas as teaching, medicine and environmental control.

Regulatory authorities are aware of the increased use and potential of computerised data systems in clinical and pre-clinical trials. The Food and Drug Administration (FDA) in the USA is already requesting that it be sent raw data in a computer-readable form to assist with its internal analysis and evaluation of data from clinical trials. The Pharmaceutical Manufacturers Association (PMA), also in the USA, has formed a joint working party with the FDA to develop the systems and procedures for a computer-assisted new drug evaluation (CANDA). Such a system, when implemented, will revolutionise the regulatory process for drug approval in the USA. Only time will tell whether or not other regulatory agencies will adopt a similar approach.

The FDA and the Department of Health (DoH) in the UK have both been active in producing guidelines for the validation of computerised data systems, with the aim of ensuring good standards of quality control and validation of computer software and hardware within the pharmaceutical industry. However, these guidelines were written specifically for pre-clinical studies and, although the principles apply equally to clinical studies, no specific guidelines are currently available for the validation of computerised data systems used in clinical trials.

I shall now consider some of the issues involved.

Data Handling

What Constitutes 'Raw Data'?

The introduction of good laboratory practice (GLP) and good clinical research practice (GCRP) has served to formalise the way studies are performed and the way in which data are recorded, stored and presented. Standard operating procedures (SOPs) are produced in order to assure the quality and integrity of data generated during a study. In pre-clinical studies, quality assurance (QA) staff are responsible for monitoring each study to ensure that facilities, equipment, personnel, methods, practices, records and controls meet GLP requirements.

In good laboratory practice, raw data are defined as 'any laboratory worksheets, records, memoranda, notes, or exact copies thereof'. GLP regulations also require that changes to raw data do not obscure the original entry. This is particularly important to enable an audit trail to be followed. The same principles are also valid for clinical studies.

Case report forms (CRFs) are recommended in the GCRP guidelines as a means of ensuring the uniformity and completeness of clinical trial data. This can be extremely important in long-term multi-centre studies to ensure that the different clinical investigators record the same information at the same time post-dose and in the same units. Such uniformity of data collection and recording is essential to ensure ease of documentation, analysis and interpretation.

The GLP requirements for data entered and stored in a computer database are no different from those for hand-recorded data. Regardless of where the raw data reside, a QA inspector must be able to review the data to assess their accuracy, validity and integrity. SOPs must be available for handling, storage, archiving, maintenance, retention and retrieval of computer generated raw data. Security issues must also be covered to ensure that raw data are protected against unauthorised access.

Computer raw data can exist on several different types of media (e.g. printout, magnetic record, microfiche, etc.). Data entered into a computer through an instrument interface are classed as raw data; data entered electronically are also classed as raw data. When a computer system is used for data collection, a back-up system must exist to ensure that data are still being recorded during periods of system failure.

Manual collection of data and their entry into a computer involves a data transcription process. Verifying the accuracy of the transcribed data is essential. Even when a set of hand-recorded data has been transcribed into a computer, the original hand-recorded data still constitute the raw data and must be kept.

The Path of the Data from Protocol to Report

Figure 18.1 shows the various pathways which can be taken by the data from protocol to report.

Once the protocol for the study is available, the case report forms can be produced. These forms should contain identifiers for all of the information and measurements which are to be obtained from a particular subject following administration of a particular treatment.

During the trial, clinical measurements can be collected in a number of ways, including manual (hand-written) recording into a notebook or onto case report forms, and automatic recording of data by an instrument. If it is required to store the data in a computer database or in files on the computer, a data entry step is required. If the data were recorded directly onto the case report forms, an additional step is needed (i.e. keyboard entry into the database). However if the data were recorded in a notebook prior to entry on the case record forms, a further data entry step is involved.

Checking the accuracy of data entered manually into a computer database is often achieved by means of a double data entry system. This allows a cross-check to be performed on the two sets of data in order to highlight any errors or inconsistencies.

If the data were recorded by an instrument (e.g. blood pressure monitor) and the instrument was not linked to a computer, a manual transcription step would be required in order to transcribe the data onto case report forms prior to entry into a computer database. However, if the instrument was linked directly to a computer and the interface procedures had been fully validated, no transcription steps would be involved. Once the data are stored in a computer database, or in appropriate files, all subsequent documentation, analysis and reporting can be performed without further data transcription.

Clearly, in those cases where manual transcription of data is necessary, extensive data checking is involved. This procedure is very time-consuming and a high error rate is likely. Automatic or semi-automatic data entry avoids this problem, but it is essential that such systems are fully validated and regularly audited.

Validation of Computerised Data Systems

Computer systems involved in the acquisition, storage, analysis and presentation of clinical and pre-clinical data must be validated in order to ensure the integrity of the procedures used.

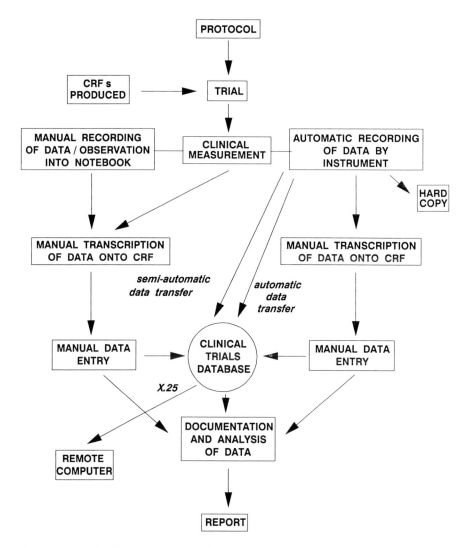

Figure 18.1. Path of data from protocol to report.

Industry Standards

A number of general industry standards and procedures for computer system development have been published by such organisations as the American National Standards Institute (ANSI), the Institute of Electrical and Electronic Engineers (IEEE) and the International Standards Organisation (ISO).

Within the pharmaceutical industry, the FDA has produced written guidelines entitled *Computerised Data Systems for Non-clinical Safety Assessment* and a technical report entitled *Software Development Activities*. The DoH have also produced an advisory leaflet on good laboratory practice entitled *The Application of GLP Principles to Computer Systems*.

Key Elements of a Computer System

Three key elements combine to make a computer system, namely hardware, software and firmware.

Hardware can be defined as 'those elements of a computer system which can be seen or physically touched', e.g. CPU, disc drive, tape drive, and terminal. Hardware deteriorates with time and hence it is essential to have some form of maintenance plan or agreement.

Regulatory authorities are less concerned with validation of the hardware aspects of a computer system. Assurances from the manufacturer, with respect to quality control, are usually sufficient. Equally they are not concerned with the validation of any instruments which produce clinical measurements. However, when the two are linked together, some form of validation is required and this is discussed later.

Software can be defined as 'programs, procedures, rules and any associated documentation pertaining to the operation of a computer system'. There are two categories of software, namely operating system software and applications software.

Operating system software controls the function and operation of the computer system (i.e. resource allocation, input–output (I/O) control and data management). This software is usually specific to the computer and its manufacturer. In the past, it was difficult to transport applications software from one machine to another owing to differences in the operating systems software. However, following years of pressure from the user, 'industry standard' operating systems are becoming commoner; for example, IBM compatibility in personal computers. Validation of the operating system software is the responsibility of the manufacturer.

Applications software accomplishes the desired task. Unlike operating system software, applications software is not usually manufacturer specific. While there is a fairly wide range of applications software available from computer manufacturers, a substantial amount of the more specialised software is written by 'third-party' companies. However, in the pharmaceutical industry during the 1970s and early 1980s, the advances in computer hardware technology were not matched by the availability of relevant applications software, leading to many 'in-house' developments. In some areas of pharmaceutical R & D this is still the case.

Where it is to be purchased, the formal validation of the software is carried out by the vendor and this is acceptable from a regulatory point of view. However, the software should be tested in the user environment to ensure that it is a 'quality product'. For 'in-house' developed software, the responsibility for validation lies with the sponsor or developer of the product. There are, however, many systems and programs in use today which were developed several years ago and which have never been formally validated. In these cases, some form of retrospective validation is necessary, although by this time the system or program will have validated itself in use.

Procedures for software validation are described below.

It should be borne in mind when considering software validation that the operating system software and the applications software must work together if a system or process is to function properly. This means that, whenever the system software of a computer is upgraded, the applications software must be tested in its new environment.

Firmware is defined as 'hardware, containing a computer program and data, that cannot be changed in its user environment'. Firmware is a hybrid of hardware and software [e.g. silicon chip, read only memory (rom), erasable programmable read only memory (eprom), etc.].

Computer Programs

A computer program is an extremely detailed set of instructions to be executed by the computer system in a predetermined order. Programs can be very complex and there may be numerous paths and branches that can be followed from instruction to instruction. The quality and validity of software can only be assured by the use of programming standards and life cycle procedures.

Programming Standards

Programming standards are essential to ensure uniformity and clarity between routines, modules and programs regardless of who wrote them; they include:

Structural standards:
- Logic flow, etc.

Coding standards:
- Naming of modules and variables.
- Conventions for designating revision levels.
- Identification of relevant programming manuals.
- Conventions on code format.
- Complexity controls (e.g. lines of code per module).

Testing standards:
- Responsibility for testing the software.
- Comment on how the test data are generated.
- Reference to who keeps test records and error logs.

Documentation:
- Helpful commenting.
- Flow charts.
- Decision trees.
- Location of documentation.
- Responsibility for documentation.

Software Life-Cycle

The software life-cycle can be likened in some ways to the development of a drug. Various stages are involved.

Requirements Phase

This stage concerns defining the requirements of the user. The clearer the user requirements are defined, the closer the result will be to that required. Discussions between the user and the project developer are an essential first step on this pathway. Following these discussions, the project developer produces a document which clearly defines the requirements specified. This document is then reviewed and approved by the user. Failure to define adequately the requirements of a project prior to coding could lead to endless modifications.

Design Phase

In this phase the requirements are converted into a specification for the program. This is where quality is built in to the program. A specification is simply a detailed set of instructions to those responsible for writing or maintaining the program. A specification should include:

- Description of activities, operations or processes which are being controlled, monitored or reported by the computer system.
- Description of the hardware to be used.
- Description of the software to be used, especially any algorithms or accuracy verification procedures.
- Description of the files created and accessed by the program and any reports generated.
- Description of all parameters to be measured and any limits which are set.
- Description of all error messages and their causes. Testing plan.
- Description of all interfaces, connections and communications between the external world, the processor and the software.
- Description of security measures to be followed.

The specification should be approved by the user and reviewed by the QA group.

Implementation Phase

The specification is now converted into a software product. At this stage the programming language is selected, coding begins and programming standards are applied. Documentation is continued throughout the project, resulting in the production of a user manual.

Test Phase

This is where the software product is evaluated to determine whether the requirements of the specification have been satisfied. The test plan (as outlined in the specification) is then implemented. The real aim of this phase is to locate as many errors as possible. This phase must be repeated following each revision of the software.

Installation Phase

The final validation of a computer program is achieved by testing the finished product in the user environment. This should also include training of the user and an assessment of his or her ability to understand and interface with the program.

Maintenance Phase

By the time this stage has been reached, the project will have been defined, specified, coded, tested and installed, and it will be fully operational. However, it may still contain 'bugs' which have not been located. Therefore, the program will need to be monitored while in use. If the operating system software is upgraded, the program will need to be retested to ensure that it still functions as expected.

Records of any changes made during this phase must be kept.

Computer Communications

Instrument to Computer Communications

In those cases where the clinical measurement is obtained using an instrument (e.g. a blood pressure monitor) and the data are transferred into a computer database, either automatically (direct capture) or semi-automatically (via floppy disc, etc.), some form of validation of the data transfer is needed. The hardware aspects of interfacing the instrument to a computer and capturing the output signal are relatively straightforward. However, the software will need to be specially 'customised', depending on the type of instrument involved and the data capture requirements.

Formal guidelines for the validation of instrument to computer communications have not yet been produced. However, it is a relatively simple process to ensure that the data output from the instrument (i.e. from a visual display or hard-copy output) is accurately transmitted to the computer by means of test data. An additional safeguard is to retain the hard-copy printout from the instrument. Standard operating procedures should contain all the necessary steps for validation.

An example of a laboratory automation system is shown in *Figure 18.2*.

Networks

Networks allow communication between different computers. They can operate over considerable distances ('wide area networks'), or can be contained within a single building or on a given site ('local area networks').

Some form of electronic communication is essential for all international companies. The advent of special modem links, such as X.25 or X.400, has made it relatively easy to use 'electronic mail'. The same technology can also be used to transmit data electronically between sites on both a local and an international level.

The electronic transfer of data forming part or all of a submission to regulatory authorities would be a relatively straightforward procedure using this technology. The FDA and the PMA have taken a step on this pathway with the CANDA project.

As with instrument-to-computer communications, there are currently no formal guidelines available for the validation of electronically transmitted data. The use of test data (as laid down in the SOP), together with a hard copy of the data, should be sufficient.

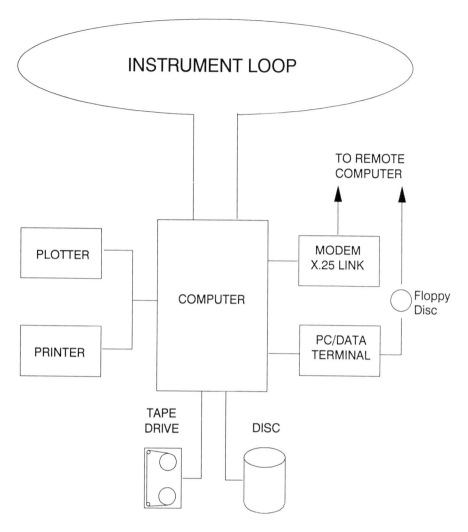

Figure 18.2. Laboratory automation system.

Conclusion

During the next five to ten years, an increased use of and reliance on computers will continue to be observed in all aspects of data handling, particularly in the areas of data capture, analysis, presentation and communication.

The advances in communications allow raw data to be transferred both within and between sites, and to regulatory authorities. In the USA, moves towards computer-assisted registration for drugs are seen as a major advance, and the validation of the software and procedures used in such data transmission is of great importance. Regulations in this area are already catching up with developments.

A quality assurance unit (QAU) has no mandated responsibility for computer system development. However, it is strongly recommended that the QAU be involved in the development of such systems in order to ensure that they meet regulatory needs. Once a computerised data system has been validated and its reliability confirmed, only periodic auditing and testing of the system would be necessary.

Development of in-house software will become a thing of the past. It will not be cost-effective for pharmaceutical companies to develop and validate their own systems. The future lies in the purchase of 'off-the-shelf' solutions which can be tailored to the customer needs. The responsibility for validation and maintenance then falls on the manufacturer. It would only be necessary for the user to test the product in the user environment.

19. Special Population Studies

B. Whiting

Introduction

The title of this article is worth looking at in a little more detail so that the contents can be more readily understood. 'Special' implies 'something particular, unusual' and, in the present context, 'exceptional in amount'. 'Population' refers to a 'number' of people, the number being unspecified at the moment, but enough to characterise a particular group of people – perhaps the target group for a particular drug. 'Studies' refers to those which primarily collect blood levels (pharmacokinetic) and to those which are concerned also with drug responses (pharmacodynamic). In the latter context, responses are regarded as both beneficial and adverse.

Before going into further detail, we should ask 'Why "special population" studies?' Advances in clinical pharmacological data analysis and experimental design have led to improvements in the control of drug therapy based on interesting statistical principles, notably Bayes Theorem. The focus of these advances is to improve the clinician's intuitive ability to select the right drug and dosage in particular circumstances so that benefit is maximised and harm minimised. Pharmacokinetic and pharmacodynamic studies may help the clinician to obtain the *a priori* information on which this control is based. Fundamentally, this information describes, in statistical terms, the variability in the pharmacokinetics and pharmacodynamics of the drug under investigation, and may also provide an explanation for this variability. The elements in this task can be seen in *Figure 19.1*, where *PD* indicates a pharmacodynamic relationship (the traditional 'dose–response' relationship), *PD'* indicates a

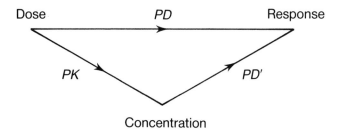

Figure 19.1. Pharmacokinetic and pharmacodynamic variabilities of a drug under investigation: the key elements.

somewhat more informative pharmacodynamic relationship which is devoid of pharmacokinetic variability, and *PK* indicates the pharmacokinetic relationship. Each of these relationships can be measured in population studies. The past ten years has seen the emergence of 'population pharmacokinetics' which deals with the variability expressed by *PK*, but this discipline is still in its infancy.

Population *versus* Traditional Data

The differences between population and traditional data reside in the fact that population studies lead to a statistical description of a (population) model and its parameters, while traditional, single subject, studies lead to the estimation of model parameters subject-by-subject. As far as the data are concerned, the usual non-linear least squares estimation procedures applied to single subject data dictate that a 'complete set' of data should be obtained (according to a specific protocol). The 'complete set' is determined by the model under investigation and, as a rule of thumb (when considering pharmacokinetic experiments), there should be $4p$ concentration–time points, where p is the number of parameters in the model. In population studies, less data per subject are permissible, but, whereas it was originally thought that *any* data could be exploited to yield population information, the current feeling is that experimental design considerations are as important in population studies as they are in traditional studies. Less data per subject *are* permissible, but the choice of the number of concentrations and their timing (and the number of subjects involved) has an important bearing on the outcome, and is still the subject of research.[1] As in any statistical description, success or failure will depend on the degree of representation of the subjects under consideration and the information content of the data collected. In population studies, the complexity of the model, in terms of the number of parameters and the way in which variability is conceived, will eventually determine the experimental protocol.

   As far as the data analysis is concerned, there are a number of non-linear least squares regression programmes which can be used to estimate parameters in traditional single-subject studies, but only the NONMEM programme[2] is readily available for population data analysis. Taking a pharmacokinetic example, where the model contains only two parameters – say clearance (*Cl*) and volume of distribution (*V*) (such as might be the case after a drug is administered intravenously) – the traditional approach would yield values of *Cl* and *V* in individual subjects (with their respective estimation errors). The population approach would yield the average values of *Cl* and *V*, and their distribution in the group of subjects analysed. In the traditional approach, the (single) subject is the unit of analysis. In the population approach, the population is the unit of analysis.

   In the above simple example, the set of population values would consist of at least:

- The mean value of *Cl*.
- The standard deviation of *Cl* – reflecting the distribution (intersubject variability) of *Cl* in the population.

- The mean value of V.
- The standard deviation of V – reflecting the distribution (intersubject variability) of V in the population.
- A (residual) value expressing the variability which has not been explained by the proposed pharmacokinetic model.

Moreover, the analysis might also seek to explain the variability in the data by proposing relationships between the kinetic parameters and measurable or observable patient features (the characteristics that describe the population) such as age, weight, sex, creatinine clearance, etc. Thus, regression models to *explain* clearance (and/or volume of distribution) may be embedded in the basic (structural) pharmacokinetic model. This is well illustrated in a recent study of the pharmacokinetics of theophylline in children[3], where theophylline clearance was shown to be determined by age, race, gender, and the presence or absence of other types of bronchodilator therapy (R_X). The regression equation had the form:

$$\log Cl = -0.23 + 0.09 . \text{AGE} + 0.3 . \text{RACE} - 0.2 . \text{SEX} - 0.4 . R_X.$$

Thus a Caucasion boy of ten, receiving no other therapy, would have a theophylline clearance estimated from the equation:

$$\log Cl = -0.23 + 0.09 \times 10 + 0 - 0 - 0$$

where RACE = 0 for white, 1 for black
SEX = 0 for male, 1 for female
R_X = 0 for nil else, 1 for other treatment.

Thus, $Cl = 2.0\,l/h$ and the intersubject variability, expressed as a coefficient of variation, had a value of 20%.

When considering pharmacodynamics, there is a choice of three fundamental equations[4], the choice depending principally on the range and extent of the data. The three possibilities are:

- The linear equation, where response is a linear function of dose or concentration, best thought of as the concentration at steady state, Cp_{ss}.
- The Langmuir equation, describing a simple sigmoid relationship.
- The Hill equation, describing a general class of sigmoid relationships.

Taking the linear equation as the simplest example, this has been used to describe the change in forced vital capacity (*FVC*) over a range of theophylline steady state concentrations in adult patients with chronic obstructive airways disease.[9] The 'population' equation had the following form:

$$FVC(L) = 0.04\,Cp_{ss} + 1.58$$
$$(\pm 0.012)\,(\pm 0.79)$$

Here the figures in parenthesis expressed the standard deviation of the slope and intercept respectively (the intercept expressing the average value and range of untreated *FVC* values). At the time this study was reported, the authors suggested that this *a priori* information on the performance of a group of patients with chronic obstructive airways disease could be used as the basis of a forecasting system; this would tailor the dose of theophylline to the anticipated response using Bayesian parameter estimation. This concept, applied in a number of therapeutic areas, still requires thorough exploration and evaluation.

Control Aspects

The concept of 'control' stems from a foundation laid by clinical pharmaco-kinetics. In a general sense, a dosage regimen chosen on the basis of population pharmacokinetic parameters will lead to a degree of uncertainty in the achievement of plasma drug concentrations. This is because of the persisting variability in the population parameters, even when they can be explained in terms of a number of covariates. This premise is well illustrated in *Figure 19.2*, where the 68% confidence interval in theophylline concentrations at steady state has been calculated on the basis of population informa-tion. The interval at 12 hours ranges from 4.5 mg/l to 17.6 mg/l with a mean

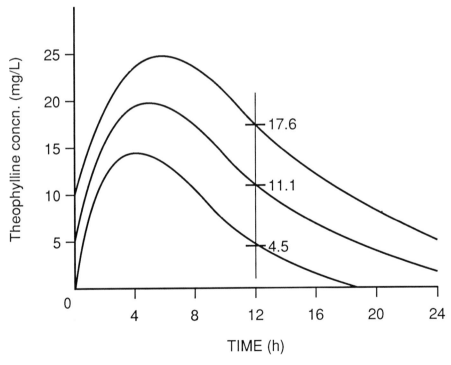

Figure 19.2. An example of the 68% confidence interval applicable to steady state theophylline concentrations when only population pharmacokinetic information is available. This interval extends from 4.5 to 17.6 mg/l (with a mean value of 11.1 mg/l) when calculated 12 h after a dose. (In this case, the dosage interval has been somewhat arbitrarily set at 24 h.)

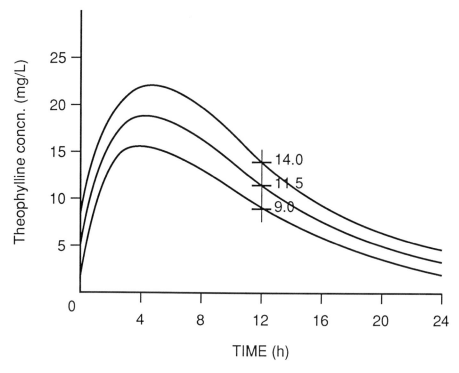

Figure 19.3. The reduction in the 68% confidence interval after two previous concentration measurements and estimation of the pharmacokinetic parameters with a Bayesian procedure. The interval at 12 h now extends from 9 to 14 mg/l, with a mean value of 11.5 mg/l.

of 11.1 mg/l, which gives a sense of the range of concentrations that may be achieved when a specific target level is sought (in this case, about 11 mg/l). This obviously leads to a hit-or-miss situation which is quite unsatisfactory in clinical practice. The uncertainty, however, can be clearly reduced by measurement of one or more concentrations in the individual. This extra information immediately shows how the individual behaves in relation to the population. Moreover, this behaviour can be characterised pharmacokineti- cally in a fairly robust statistical way using Bayesian parameter estimation[7], allowing a new confidence interval to be calculated, as illustrated in *Figure 19.3*. Here, two (previous) concentration measurements ('feedbacks') have been used to revise the initial uncertainty, generated by purely population information, to yield a new 68% confidence interval extending from 9–14 mg/l, a considerable improvement on *Figure 19.2*. The computation involved has shifted the *a priori* values of the population pharmacokinetic parameters to new *a posteriori* values, each of which may now be known with more certainty (i.e. with smaller standard deviations) in the individual. Such an approach has made a tremendous impact on the interpretation of 'blood levels' in clinical pharmacokinetic practice, and can be readily implemented on microcomputers.[6]

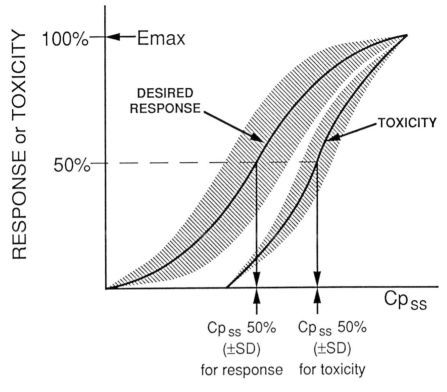

Figure 19.4. Diagrammatic illustration of the variability (shaded areas) surrounding mean population pharmacodynamic curves for both the desired response and toxicity of a drug. E_{max} indicates the maximum response (desired or toxic) to the drug, and the Cp_{ss} 50% values are those steady state concentrations associated with 50% desired response or toxicity. Response and toxicity are both scaled to a maximum of 100%.

The 'target blood level' objective, however, has its limitations. It is rooted to the idea that there is a reasonably unwavering relationship between concentration and response across patients, and, when considering an individual, this may not be the case. The pharmacodynamic relationship may also be subject to greater or lesser variability, and this may confound the relatively simplistic concept of the 'therapeutic range' (for *all* patients). A more attractive idea, in some therapeutic circumstances, is to think in terms of a range of concentrations *in the individual* which will maximise benefit and minimise harm. This is obviously the aim of all rational therapy, and its implementation would represent an interesting extension to traditional pharmacokinetics. The important difference, in terms of the extension, would be the formal mathematical and statistical inclusion of beneficial and adverse drug response data, enabling the change of benefit in relation to harm (the 'utility') across a range of concentrations to be calculated.[5] As in Bayesian pharmacokinetic parameter estimation, this would require equivalent information on the nature and statistical distribution of pharmacodynamic parameters, and calls for 'special' population pharmacodynamic studies. Indeed,

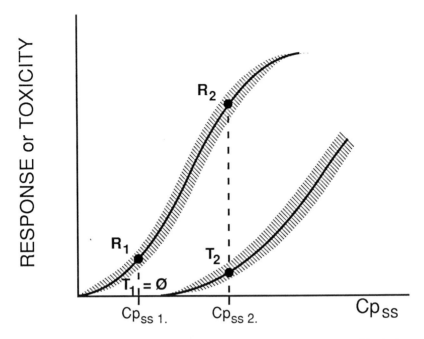

Figure 19.5. Diagrammatic representation of the reduction in variability (shaded areas) associated with desired response and toxicity when concentration, response and toxicity information unique to the individual is used to revise the initial population pharmacodynamic parameters by a Bayesian procedure. R_1 and R_2 are response measurements at two Cp_{ss} levels, Cp_{ss1} and Cp_{ss2}. T_1 is a toxicity assessment at Cp_{ss1}, (nil in this case) and T_2 is the level of toxicity assessed at Cp_{ss2}. The solid curves now characterise the mean expected performance of the individual in pharmacodynamic terms.

with a view to the introduction of this approach, designs for such studies are now being discussed and developed.[8]

The possible outcome of a population pharmacodynamic study, based on sigmoid relationships for both the desired response and the associated toxic effect, is illustrated in *Figure 19.4*. If the shaded areas represent the variability in (desired) response and toxicity (derived, for example, from NONMEM estimates of the variability in the various pharmacodynamic parameters), this provides the *a priori* information necessary for subsequent Bayesian parameter estimation, facilitated by measurements which will characterise the individual. In this case, the measurements will consist of the response (if any) and toxicity (if any) which are achieved by a particular (steady state) concentration. Having previously defined the *a priori* nature of the pharmacodynamics, the unique observations relevant to the individual then lead to a set of *a posteriori* pharmacodynamic parameters which allow calculation of the new, less variable pharmacodynamic relationships, shown in *Figure 19.5*, which now characterise the individual. Moreover, the difference between (desired) response and toxicity, i.e response *minus* toxicity, evaluated across the permissible concentration range, provides an estimate of

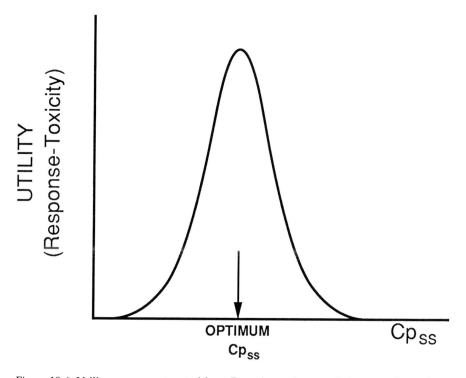

Figure 19.6. Utility curve constructed from Bayesian estimates of pharmacodynamics similar to those in *Figure 19.5*. The difference between response and toxicity across the permissible steady state concentration range has been calculated. The concentration associated with the 'peak' of this curve maximises response and minimises toxicity.

'utility' (*Figure 19.6*) where the 'optimum concentration' is that concentration associated with the peak of the utility curve. Obviously, if the peak is flattened (and prolonged) this will provide an indication of the optimum concentration range in the individual.

There has been no formal implementation of this approach yet, but its appeal is obvious in circumstances where the balance between benefit and harm is critical and depends largely on the choice of dose (and hence the achievement of optimum concentrations). An obvious example is the maintenance of the viability of organ grafts with cyclosporin in the face of potential toxicity and/or rejection.

The approach to population pharmacodynamics is rather more complex than that to population pharmacokinetics. Experimental design is of paramount importance and a number of crucial issues have to be addressed. These include:

- The type and number of patients.
- The heterogeneity they exhibit.
- The inclusion of placebos in treatment/study schedules.
- The range and order of doses.

- The clinical relevance and number of response measurements.
- The ability to identify and successfully quantitate adverse effects.
- The errors involved in all response measurements.
- The number, timing and accuracy of concentration measurements.

These are interesting and challenging issues which will require thorough exploration, but a start has been made with the suggestion that a dose–escalation design should be used when studies are being considered for subsequent population pharmacodynamic analysis.[8] This design allows all subjects to contribute varying amounts of information to the population dose, or concentration, response and toxicity curves, and facilitates the type of data analysis which is possible with the NONMEM software. Success depends on information about the entire shape of the dose–response curve (the Cp_{ss} 50% and E_{max} must be well defined) and about the inter- and intra-subject variability in the dynamic parameters. The repeated nature of the observations (within any subject) in a dose–escalation design provides the correct framework for this analysis.

Conclusion

Population studies applied to pharmacokinetic data are now seen as extremely useful tools in drug development and in clinical pharmacokinetic practice. Understanding and adjusting for pharmacokinetic variability is an integral part of rational therapeutics. The introduction of Bayesian concepts into this arena has proved invaluable, and there is no reason why these developments should not now be extended to assessments of drug response. As far as drug development, and the pharmaceutical industry, is concerned, it will be a good day when the epithet 'special' is dropped from population studies.

References

[1] Al-Banna, M.K., Kelman, A.W., and Whiting, B. Experimental design and efficient parameter estimation in population pharmacokinetics. *J. Pharmacokinet. Biopharma.*, **18**, 347–60, 1990.
[2] Beal, S.L. and Sheiner, L.B. *NONMEM Users Guide*, Parts I–VI, Division of Clinical Pharmacology, University of California, San Francisco. 1979–89.
[3] Driscoll, M.S., Ludden, T.M., Casto, D.T., and Littlefield, L.C. Evaluation of theophylline pharmacokinetics in a paediatric population using mixed effects models. *J. Pharmacokinet. Biopharma.*, **17**, 141–68, 1989.
[4] Holford, N.H.G. and Sheiner, L.B. Understanding the dose–effect relationship: clinical application of pharmacokinetic–pharmacodynamic models. *Clin. Pharmacokinet.*, **6**, 429–53, 1981.
[5] Kelman, A.W. and Whiting, B. A Bayesian approach to the utility of drug therapy. *Biomedical Measurement Informatics and Control*, **20**, 170–5, 1988.
[6] Kelman, A.W., Whiting, B., and Bryson, S.M. OPT: a package of computer programs for parameter optimisation in clinical pharmacokinetics. *Br. J. Clin. Pharmacol.*, **14**, 247–56, 1982.

[7] Sheiner, L.B., Beal, S.L., Rosenberg, B., and Marathe, V.V. Forecasting individual pharmacokinetics. *Clin. Pharmacol. Therapeut.*, **26**, 294–305, 1979.

[8] Sheiner, L.B., Beal, S.L., and Sambol, N.C. Study designs for dose ranging. *Clin. Pharmacol. Therapeut.*, **46**, 63–77, 1989.

[9] Whiting, B., Kelman, A.W., and Struthers, A.D. Prediction of response to theophylline in chronic bronchitis. *Br. J. Clin. Pharmacol.*, **17**, 1–8, 1984.

20. Detection and Collection of Adverse Drug Reactions

A. Breckenridge

Introduction

In this chapter I do not intend to discuss methods of adverse drug reaction, detection and collection, or consider the relative advantages and disadvantages of such techniques as spontaneous reporting schemes, cohort and control studies. Rather I propose to assume a broad understanding of these methods and to discuss, instead, with some recent examples, how investigation of adverse events is being used to help us understand the clinical and scientific basis of drug toxicity.

The history of drug regulation is in fact the history of drug safety. For centuries, therapeutic agents showing no good evidence of efficacy but manifest toxicity have been administered to man. By the early nineteenth century, the only groups of drugs with specific therapeutic actions known to man were the alkaloids and glycosides, such as digitalis. Inhalational anaesthetics, early analgesics and barbiturates followed, but there were still many botanical substances of uncertain purity sold as drugs and adulteration remained a problem. The Adulteration Act (originally applied to food and drink alone, and only later to therapeutic substances) became law in Britain in 1860, and the first *British Pharmacopoeia* was published in 1864, although this contained very few pure substances which had a specific therapeutic action. The first attempt to control the retailing of poisons was by the Pharmacy Act of 1868.

One of the strangest stories of drug regulation in this country concerns the report of the Select Committee on Patent Medicines, which was printed on 4 August 1914, the day World War I broke out. This report recommended, among other things, the creation of a Medicines Commission, the delegation of matters of drug regulation to a separate division of the Department of Health, an annual fee for the registration of drugs, and empowering the Government Chemist to test for drug purity. Because of the outbreak of war, this report was not followed up. If it had been implemented, the UK would have had a system of drug regulation in place before any of the modern therapeutic agents were created, and one which it ultimately took another fifty years to create. As Mann says, 'It is not altogether fanciful to look on the children of the thalidomide disaster as late and unwitting victims of World War I.'[6]

Thalidomide, of course, plays an important part in the history of UK drug regulation. More than 10,000 deformed children (some 500 in the UK) were born to mothers who had taken thalidomide in early pregnancy, and the realisation of the imperfections of drug regulation led to the establishment in 1964 of the Committee on Safety of Drugs, chaired by Sir Derrick Dunlop. This committee was more concerned with drug safety than drug efficacy; Dunlop, writing in 1966, noted: 'The Committee's remit does not impose on it any responsibility to consider efficacy, except insofar as safety is concerned. The Committee's clearance of a drug for marketing does not necessarily imply its approval of it as a remedy.'[4]

All this changed with the Medicines Act of 1968 which became law in 1972. For the first time, drug efficacy and quality, as well as safety, had to be taken into account in licensing a therapeutic agent in the UK. With this, the concept of the balance between risk and benefit became important in all licensing activities.

Basis of Adverse Drug Reactions

Assessment of the basis of adverse drug reactions has changed considerably over the years as our understanding of pharmacology has improved. One of the first attempts to classify adverse drug reactions was by Brodie in 1968.[2] The first type could be understood from knowledge of the physiological control systems on which drugs acted and could largely be predicted from animal studies. The second type, which was less predictable, was thought to involve structural and biochemical damage to the cell. This classification is not unreasonable, considering how fragmentary, at that time, was our understanding of such important aspects of clinical pharmacology as inter-individual differences in drug metabolism and receptor pharmacology.

By 1977, pharmacological knowledge had obviously increased, and Rawlins and Thompson[8] were able to make a more comprehensive attempt to classify adverse drug reactions – a classification still used widely today (*Table 20.1*). Under this classification, type A adverse reactions broadly corresponded to the first type described by Brodie, in that they were largely predictable from animal pharmacology and were dose related. Type A reactions occurred frequently, but had a low mortality, while type B reactions (presumed to have largely an immunological basis) occurred relatively infrequently, but with a high mortality resulting. The basis of type B reactions remained somewhat ill defined, in keeping with our understanding of immunological events in the late 1970s. The merit of this classification over Brodie's earlier attempt is that it clearly takes into account our burgeoning understanding of inter-individual differences in all aspects of pharmacokinetics.

The third classification of adverse drug reactions which I cite is that given by Grahame-Smith and Aronson in 1984 (*Table 20.2*).[5] Types 1 and 2 correspond almost exactly with Rawlins and Thompson's type A and B effects, although their basis is slightly more explicit. Two other types have been added: 'long-term effects' and 'delayed effects'. It is known that adaptive changes occur in response to drug therapy and can form the basis of adverse reactions. Examples include the tolerance to, and the physical dependence on, narcotic analgesics, and tardive dyskinesias in some patients

Table 20.1. Classification of adverse drug reactions.[8]

Type A:
  Due to abnormality in:
  1. Pharmacokinetic factors
  2. Pharmacodynamic alteration in sensitivity of target organs due to
       • genetic factors
       • disease

Type B:
  Due to abnormality in:
  1. Pharmacokinetic factors
       • drug, e.g. additive
       • patient, e.g. production of abnormal metabolite
  2. Pharmacodynamic alteration in sensitivity of target organ due to:
       • genetic factors
       • immunological response

Table 20.2. Classification of adverse drug reactions.[5]

Dose-related (Type A or augmented):
  1. Pharmaceutical variation
  2. Pharmacokinetic variations
       • pharmacogenetic variations
       • hepatic disease
       • renal disease
       • cardiac disease
       • thyroid disease
  3. Pharmacodynamic variation
       • hepatic disease
       • altered fluid and electrolyte balance

Non-dose-related (Type B or bizarre)
  1. Immunological reactions
  2. Pharmacogenetic variations

Long-term effects.
Delayed effects.

---

on neuroleptic therapy. Furthermore, the withdrawal of such drugs as the centrally acting barbiturates, benzodiazepines and the antihypertensive cloni-dine, can provoke severe clinical problems. Withdrawal of corticosteroids (after long-term usage), and of anticonvulsants and beta-adrenoceptor block-ing agents (when used in patients with ischaemic heart disease) must be done with great care to avoid danger to the patient. The basis of other long-term effects, such as retinopathy caused by chloroquine and renal damage caused by analgesics, remain poorly understood. In the fourth group of adverse reactions, delayed effects include carcinogenesis and effects on reproduction. This is still a confused and difficult area, and how far these effects can be predicted from the types of animal studies which drug regulatory authorities still require is the subject of continuing debate.

Thus it is clear that, together with our understanding of human pharmacology, our comprehension of the basis of adverse drug reactions has also progressed. This can be illustrated by considering three examples of adverse reactions from the current literature. These indicate how modern methods of clinical measurement have increased our ability to detect and to understand the basis of adverse drug reactions.

Cardiac Arrhythmias Produced by Antiarrhythmic Agents

It has been suspected for many years that antiarrhythmic drugs can themselves be pro-arrhythmic. The frequency of this type of adverse event was always believed to be low, and the benefit of administering antiarrhythmic agents prophylactically to patients with no history of sustained arrhythmia was held to be much greater than any risks incurred. The Cardiac Arrhythmia Suppression Trial (CAST) gives the lie to this supposition.[3]

The aim of CAST was to evaluate the effect of antiarrhythmic therapy with the class I agents encainide, flecainide or moricizine in patients with asymptomatic ventricular arrhythmias after myocardial infarction. The study was carefully conducted, being placebo-controlled, randomised and multicentre based. By March 1989, 1727 patients had been studied and were available for a ten-month evaluation. In that part of the trial referable to encainide and flecainide (730 patients), a comparison with 725 placebo-treated patients showed a significantly poorer survival ($p = 0.0003$) in the drug treated patients (56 deaths compared to 22).[3]

Both encainide and flecainide are in part eliminated by metabolic clearance and in part unchanged in urine. The hepatic metabolism of flecainide is subject to genetic polymorphism and this corresponds to that governing debrisoquine and sparteine, i.e. it is governed by cytochrome $P450_{DB}$. Extensive metabolisers of flecainide are known to have a higher oral drug clearance than poor metabolisers. Interest now lies in defining the metabolic status of those subjects who incur an arrhythmia while taking flecainide. It has been hypothesised that these might be of the poor metaboliser (PM) phenotype, with resulting higher drug concentrations after a standard dose. However, while this has been suggested, it is difficult to prove because the arrhythmia incurred may be fatal.[7] Anecdotal evidence, however, supports the hypothesis. This does illustrate the main thesis of this paper, namely that an understanding of the modern concepts of pharmacology may help our assessment of adverse drug reactions.

Toxicity of Mianserin

Mianserin is a widely used antidepressant, but it causes agranulocytosis and hepatotoxicity with a frequency varying between 1 in 10,000 and 1 in 50,000 in various populations. The basis of these effects is poorly understood and has been considered as typical type B reactions (Rawlins and Thompson) or type 2 reactions (Grahame-Smith and Aronson). The work of Park and his colleagues[9] has been directed at understanding better the basis of its toxicity.

Park has adapted the methods of Spielberg et al.[10] to design a cytotoxicity assay. The hypothesis underlying this work is that many adverse effects may not be caused by the parent drug, but by unstable and toxic metabolites which are difficult to identify. By using an incubation technique in which the drug is exposed, under ideal conditions, to a complete drug metabolising system including human liver, these metabolites may be generated. The system is housed in a multicompartmental apparatus, one section of which contains 'target' cells in which the toxicity is manifest. Mianserin and human liver are placed in one compartment, separated by a semi-permeable membrane from human lymphocytes. The viability of the lymphocytes can be measured after a fixed period of exposure to drug metabolite as described elsewhere. Park has clearly shown[9] that the toxicity of mianserin for human lymphocytes can be demonstrated only when human liver is used and not liver from other species. Furthermore, increasing glutathione or ascorbate concentrations significantly decreases drug toxicity by decreasing the concentration of active metabolite generated.

This type of study will shed increasing light on previously poorly understood examples of drug toxicity, and its application to other examples is currently being explored.

Hormone Replacement Therapy (HRT) and breast cancer

Much effort has gone into investigating a possible relationship between the use of HRT and the development of breast cancer. The literature is extensive and contradictory. A recent study by Bergqvist et al.[1] addressed the subject again. In a large controlled study, involving some 23,244 Swedish women, 35 years or older, who were followed up for an average of 5.7 years, some 253 cases of breast cancer were identified. A relative risk of some 4.4 in women given HRT for between 73 and 108 months was discovered, compared to controls (95% confidence limits 0.9–22.4). It is interesting to note public reaction to this study. Commentators noted the wide confidence limits cited and analysed the effect of HRT in terms of risk and benefit. While acknowledging that there may be a slight increase in the risk of developing breast cancer (and this is still debated), most experts considered that the benefits afforded by HRT – the decrease in osteoporotic bone fractures, and protection from endometrial cancer, ischaemic heart disease and perhaps stroke – outweigh any risk of breast cancer increase.

This illustrates the point that all forms of drug toxicity must not only be assessed in terms of risk, but must also take account of the benefit that the therapy may confer.

Conclusion

Current methods of detecting adverse drug reactions must be modified in the light of modern pharmacological knowledge and this will affect our methods of classifying these reactions. New types of molecule, such as therapeutic peptides, will create difficult situations for assessing drug toxicity, and methods must be devised to cope with this. Drug toxicity must be considered as an integral part of drug action. As we understand more of one, so we will understand more of the other.

References

[1] Bergkvist, L., Adami, H.O., Persson, I., Hoover, R., and Schainer, C. The risk of breast cancer after estrogen and estrogen-progestin replacement. *N. Eng. J. Med.*, **321**, 293–7, 1989.

[2] Brodie, B.B. The mechanisms of adverse drug reactions. In *Mechanisms of Drug Toxicity*, H. Raskova (ed), Vol. 4, pp 23–47, Pergamon Press, Oxford, 1968.

[3] Cardiac Arrhythmia Suppression Trial (CAST) Investigators. Preliminary report: effect of encainide and flecainide on mortality in a randomised trial of arrhythmia suppression after myocardial infarction. *N. Eng. J. Med.*, **321**, 406–12, 1989.

[4] Dunlop, D. The assessment of the safety of drugs and the role of government in their control. *J. Clin. Pharmacol.*, **1**, 184–92, 1967.

[5] Grahame-Smith, D.G. and Aronson, J.K. Adverse reactions to drugs. In *Oxford Textbook of Clinical Pharmacology*, Oxford University Press, Oxford, pp 132–57, 1984.

[6] Mann, R. *Modern Drug Usage. An Enquiry into Historical Principles*. MTP Press, Lancaster, UK, 1984.

[7] Mikus, G., Gross, A.S., Beckmann, J., Hertrampf, R., Gundert-Remy, U., and Eichelbaum, M. The influence of the sparteine-debrisoquine phenotype on the disposition of flecainide. *Clin. Pharmacol. Therapeut.*, **45**, 562–7, 1989.

[8] Rawlins, M.D. and Thompson, J.W. Mechanisms of adverse drug reactions. In *Textbook of Adverse Drug Reactions*, D.M. Davies, (ed), Oxford University Press, Oxford, pp 12–38, 1977.

[9] Riley, R.J., Lambert, C., Kitteringham, N.R., and Park, B.K. A stereochemical investigation of the cytotoxicity of mianserin metabolites *in vitro*. *Br. J. Clin. Pharmacol.*, **27**, 823–30, 1989.

[10] Spielberg, S.P. Acetaminophen toxicity in human lymphocytes *in vitro*. *J. Pharmacy Pharmacol.*, **213**, 395–8, 1980.

Index